KU-678-853

contents

ACKNOWLEDGEMENTS

The *BESTMEDICINE Simple Guides* team is very grateful to a number of people who have made this project possible. In particular we'd like to thank Anne Taylor, Jane Cassidy, Caroline Delasalle and Amelie (5 months). Thank you to Ben for his endless enthusiasm, energy and creativity, to Molly (7) and George (5) and of course to Hetta. Julie and Rob who went far beyond the call of duty and Julie's ability to put pages together for hours on end was hugely inspiring.

A Simple Guide to your Health Service

Emma Catherall   Co-ordinator

Advisory Panel

Richard Stevens	GP
Julieanne Jeffries	Specialist asthma nurse
David Halpin	Respiratory specialist
Michael Gum	Pharmacist
John Chater	Binley's health and care information specialist *www.binleys.com*

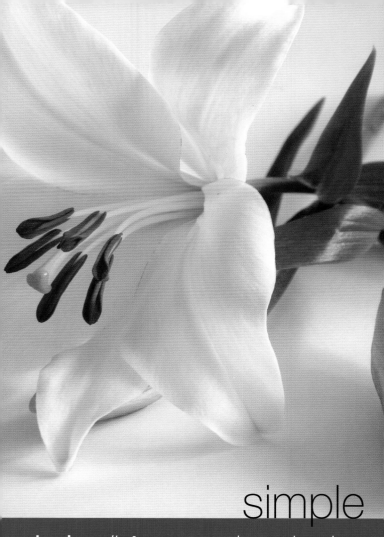

simple

simple *adj*. **1.** easy to understand or do: *a simple problem*. **2.** plain; unadorned: *a simple dress*. **3.** Not combined or complex: *a simple mechanism*. **4.** Unaffected or unpretentious: *although he became famous he remained a simple man*. **5.** sincere; frank: *a simple explanation was readily accepted*. **6**. (*prenominal*) without additions or modifications: *the witness told the simple truth*.

ABOUT THE AUTHOR

ELEANOR BULL

Eleanor graduated from King's College London with a BSc Honours degree in Pharmacology and then completed a PhD in Neuroscience at the University of Nottingham. As well as publishing her own research work internationally, Eleanor has written for numerous publications in the BESTMEDICINE *series. She now lives in the West of Ireland.*

ABOUT THE EDITOR

DAVID PRICE

David is a practising GP and Professor of Primary Care Respiratory Medicine at the University of Aberdeen. He is an active member of the General Practice Airways group (GPIAG) and the International Primary Care Respiratory Group (IPCRG).

FOREWORD

TRISHA MACNAIR
Doctor and BBC Health Journalist

Getting involved in managing your own medical condition – or helping those you love or care for to manage theirs – is a vital step towards keeping as healthy as possible. Whilst doctors, nurses and the rest of your healthcare team can help you with expert advice and guidance, nobody knows your body, your symptoms and what is right for *you* as well as you do.

There is no long-term (chronic) medical condition or illness that I can think of where the person concerned has absolutely no influence at all on their situation. The way you choose to live your life, from the food you eat to the exercise you take, will impact upon your disease, your well-being and how able you are to cope. You are in charge!

Being involved in making choices about your treatment helps you to feel in control of your problems, and makes sure you get the help that you really need. Research clearly shows that when people living with a chronic illness take an active role in looking after themselves, they can bring about significant improvements in their illness and vastly improve the quality of life they enjoy. Of course, there may be occasions when you feel particularly unwell and it all seems out of your control. Yet most of the time there are plenty of things that you can do in order to reduce the negative effects that your condition can have on your life. This way you feel as good as possible and may even be able to alter the course of your condition.

So how do you gain the confidence and skills to take an active part in managing your condition, communicate with health professionals and work through sometimes worrying and emotive issues? The answer is to become better informed. Reading about your problem, talking to others who have been through similar experiences and hearing what the experts have to say will all help to build-up your understanding and help you to take an active role in your own health care.

BESTMEDICINE Simple Guides provide an invaluable source of help, giving you the facts that you need in order to understand the key issues and discuss them with your doctors and other professionals involved in your care. The information is presented in an accessible way but without neglecting the important details. Produced independently and under the guidance of medical experts *A Simple Guide to Asthma* is an evidence-based, balanced and up-to-date review that I hope you will find enables you to play an active part in the successful management of your condition.

what happens normally?

HOW DO OUR LUNGS WORK?

In order to understand what's going on when you have asthma, it is important to first understand what happens in our lungs normally.

WHAT HAPPENS WHEN WE BREATHE?

When we breathe in, the air travels down our windpipe, or trachea, which splits into two tubes called bronchi (singular bronchus) and these divert the air into each lung. Inside the lungs, the bronchus divides further into smaller and smaller tubes, the smallest of which are called the bronchioles. From the bronchioles, the air passes into tiny air sacs, or alveoli. This is the part of our lungs where the exchange of carbon dioxide for oxygen, their most important function, takes place.

There are 300 million or so alveoli in our lungs. If they were spread out they would cover a piece of ground roughly the size of a tennis court.

When they are full of air, the alveoli inflate like tiny balloons. Alveoli are smaller than grains of salt and there are about 300 million of them in the lungs. A cross-section through a normal lung looks a bit like a pink sponge.

Breathing is something we don't normally have to think about too much. The entire process is co-ordinated by our brain, which controls a number of powerful 'breathing muscles' that are located in the ribcage. These are:

10,000 litres of air move in and out of our lungs every day.

- the intercostal muscles (surround the ribs)
- the diaphragm (a dome shaped muscle that separates the chest from the abdomen).

Breathing in

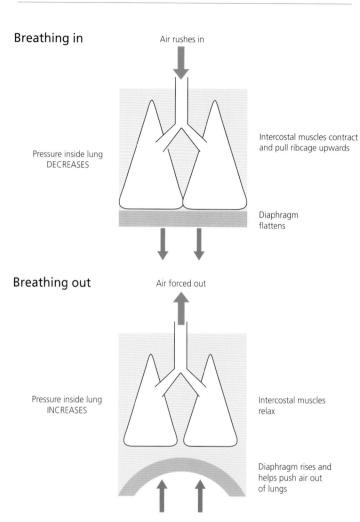

Air rushes in

Pressure inside lung
DECREASES

Intercostal muscles contract
and pull ribcage upwards

Diaphragm
flattens

Breathing out

Air forced out

Pressure inside lung
INCREASES

Intercostal muscles
relax

Diaphragm rises and
helps push air out
of lungs

THE MOVEMENT OF AIR THROUGH THE LUNGS IS CONTROLLED BY THE
DIAPHRAGM AND THE INTERCOSTAL MUSCLES.

WHY IS OXYGEN AND CARBON DIOXIDE EXCHANGE SO IMPORTANT?

By exchanging carbon dioxide for oxygen, our lungs enable us to live. Once inside the body, we use oxygen to unlock energy from food.

The surfaces of the alveoli are covered with narrow blood vessels called capillaries. Because they are so narrow, the oxygen we breathe is passed directly from the alveoli into the bloodstream and pumped all over our bodies by the heart. At the same time that oxygen is transferred into our bloodstream, carbon dioxide is taken out of our bloodstream. So, the air we breathe in contains oxygen and the air we breathe out contains carbon dioxide.

The air we breathe in is made up of 78% nitrogen, 21% oxygen, 0.03% carbon dioxide and 0.5% water.

KEY TERMS ASSOCIATED WITH THE LUNGS

	What is it?
Alveoli	Tiny air sacs that inflate like balloons when full of air.
Bloodstream	The blood flowing through the circulatory system (i.e. veins, arteries and capillaries).
Bronchi	Large air tubes that lead from the trachea to the lungs.
Bronchiole	Smaller air tube.
Capillaries	Tiny blood vessels with very thin walls. Where gas exchange takes place.
Carbon dioxide	Waste gas produced by the body.
Oxygen	Gas in the air that is vital for life.
Smooth muscle	Muscle that controls the size of the airways. Works automatically without your being aware of it.
Trachea (windpipe)	Tube through which air flows from outside the body into the bronchi.

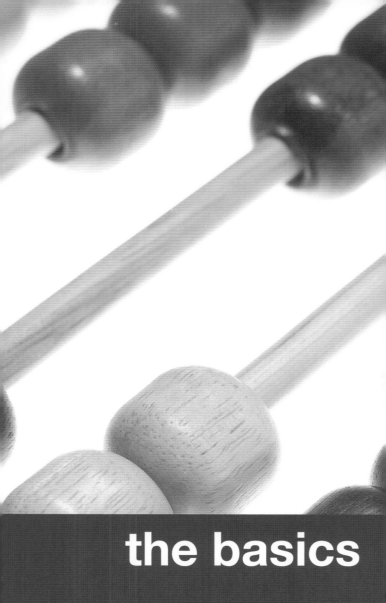

the basics

ASTHMA – THE BASICS

Asthma is a long-term condition that affects the airways – the small tubes that carry air in and out of the lungs. If you have asthma your airways become inflamed and narrow, and you experience difficulty in breathing.

In asthma, the airways narrow and this makes breathing difficult. A number of changes occur in the airways of a person with asthma, all of which can be reversed with the correct treatment. In asthma:

- the linings of the airways swell
- plugs of mucus and damaged cells block parts of the airways
- the nose is irritated and may become blocked
- the muscles of the airways tighten.

An allergy is a reaction that occurs when the immune system mistakenly identifies a normally harmless substance as damaging to the body.

■ Asthma is an inflammatory disease. The airways of people with asthma are usually red and inflamed.

■ Asthma is strongly linked to allergy. Allergies can make asthma worse. However, not all people with asthma have allergies, and not all people with allergies have asthma.

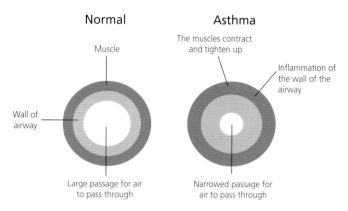

Normal	Asthma

Muscle

The muscles contract
and tighten up

Inflammation of
the wall of the
airway

Wall of
airway

Large passage for air
to pass through

Narrowed passage for
air to pass through

THE CHANGES TO THE AIRWAYS THAT OCCUR IN ASTHMA.

WHAT IS AN ASTHMA ATTACK?

During an asthma attack, the changes in the
lungs suddenly become much worse, the
airway openings become smaller and the flow
of air through them is drastically reduced,
which can make breathing extremely difficult.

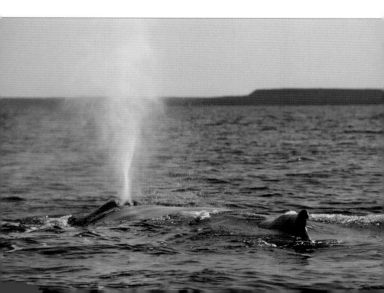

SYMPTOMS

The changes in the airways that occur in asthma mean that it requires much more of an effort to move air in and out of the lungs. This can lead to the following symptoms:

- breathlessness
- chest tightness
- wheezing
- coughing (more often in children than in adults).

Not everybody will experience these symptoms. Some people experience them from time to time; a few people may experience these symptoms all the time. The symptoms of asthma often worsen at night or after coming into contact with asthma triggers.

TRIGGERS

An allergen is a substance that causes asthma symptoms by bringing about an allergic reaction.

Although in asthma the underlying airway inflammation is always there, asthma can be worsened, or triggered, by a number of factors. There are two types of asthma triggers – allergens and irritants.

- Common asthma allergens include pollen, animals and house-dust mites.
- Common asthma irritants include cold air, cigarette smoke and chemical fumes.

An irritant is a substance that causes asthma symptoms by aggravating the airways.

Keeping a diary of the times and circumstances when your asthma is worse can help you and your doctor pinpoint exactly what your asthma triggers are. Once you have identified your asthma triggers, you can take steps to deal with them.

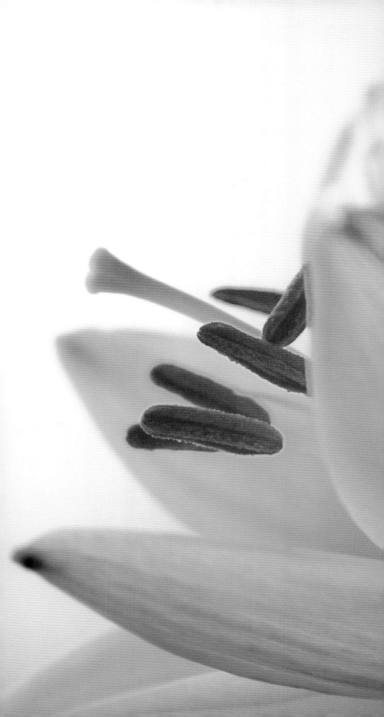

A peak flow meter measures how fast you can blow out air after taking a deep breath.

DIAGNOSING ASTHMA

Asthma is usually diagnosed on the basis of 'lung function' tests – which monitor how well your lungs are working – and the symptoms you describe to your GP. Your doctor will use a small plastic device called a peak flow meter to measure how fast you can blow air out of your lungs.

Your doctor will ask you about your symptoms and listen to your chest with a stethoscope to find out how well your airways are working. There are a number of clues that will alert a doctor to asthma, including:

- changes in the severity of your symptoms
- coming and going of symptoms
- worsening of symptoms at night
- worsening of symptoms by asthma triggers.

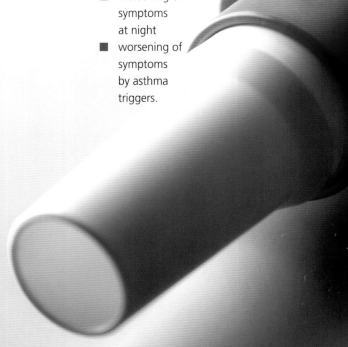

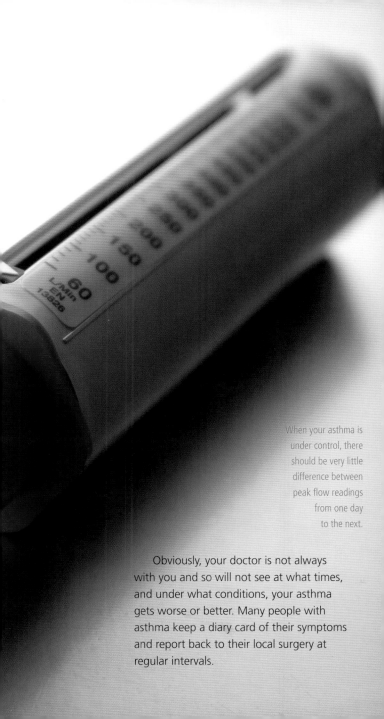

150
100
60
L/Min
EN
13826

When your asthma is under control, there should be very little difference between peak flow readings from one day to the next.

Obviously, your doctor is not always with you and so will not see at what times, and under what conditions, your asthma gets worse or better. Many people with asthma keep a diary card of their symptoms and report back to their local surgery at regular intervals.

MANAGING ASTHMA

Because asthma is a long-term, or chronic, condition it requires continuous management. Although there is no cure for asthma, there are some very effective asthma treatments that can help to control your symptoms. Your doctor or asthma nurse specialist will give you a personal asthma plan to help you keep track of what medication you need to take and what to do in the event of an emergency. An asthma management plan aims to:

- reduce your asthma symptoms
- limit the amount of medication you have to take
- prevent emergency visits to hospital
- improve your asthma-related quality of life.

There are two main kinds of asthma medication that your doctor may prescribe: drugs which, if taken regularly, may prevent an asthma attack from occurring in the first place ('**preventers**') and drugs that relieve the symptoms of an attack ('**relievers**') should one occur.

Preventers reduce inflammation and make your lungs less senstive to asthma triggers.

Relievers help to relax the airways so that they open up and allow you to breathe more easily.

FIVE STEPS TO ASTHMA CONTROL

1. Ask your doctor to prepare a written personal asthma management plan.

2. Take medications as prescribed by your doctor.

3. Be aware of the factors that make your asthma worse.

4. Learn to recognise when your symptoms are getting worse and keep a diary of these times.

5. Know what to do if your asthma worsens or if you have an asthma attack.

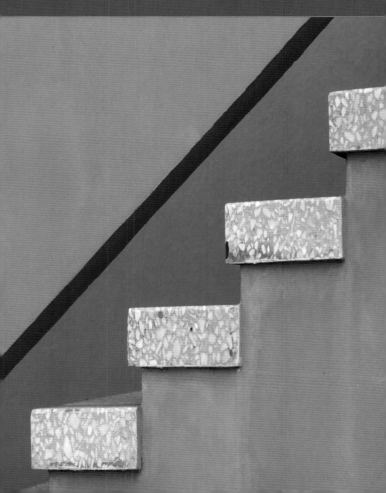

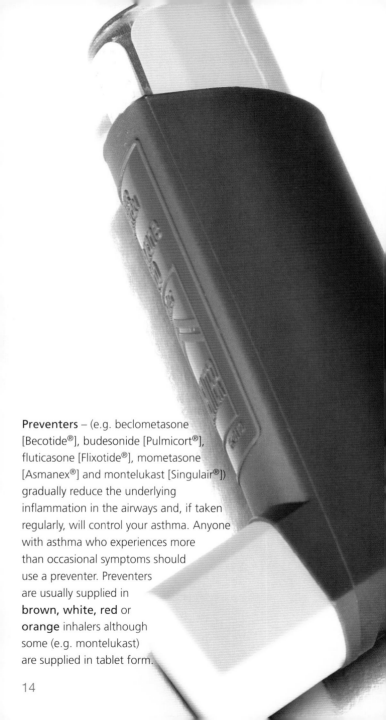

Preventers – (e.g. beclometasone [Becotide®], budesonide [Pulmicort®], fluticasone [Flixotide®], mometasone [Asmanex®] and montelukast [Singulair®]) gradually reduce the underlying inflammation in the airways and, if taken regularly, will control your asthma. Anyone with asthma who experiences more than occasional symptoms should use a preventer. Preventers are usually supplied in **brown, white, red** or **orange** inhalers although some (e.g. montelukast) are supplied in tablet form.

14

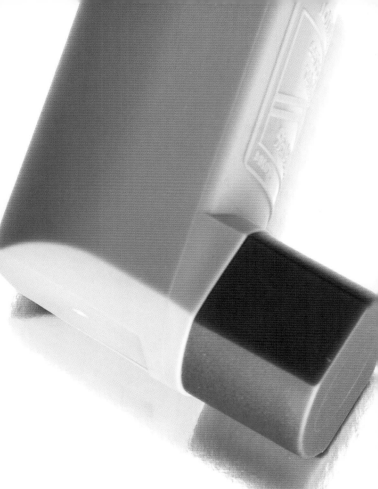

Relievers – (e.g. salbutamol [Ventolin®], terbutaline [Bricanyl®], formoterol [Foradil®, Oxis®] and salmeterol [Serevent®]) rapidly reverse the narrowing of the airways that occurs during an asthma attack. Relievers are usually supplied in **blue** or **grey** inhalers.

Bearing in mind how similar some of the symptoms of asthma and hay fever (allergic rhinitis) are, it is often a good idea to treat both conditions at the same time. People with asthma may find that their symptoms are improved after taking hay fever medications like antihistamines (e.g. Neoclarityn®, Pirteze® and Telfast®) and corticosteroid nasal sprays (e.g. Beconase®, Flixonase®).

As well as taking drugs, there are a number of changes you can make to your lifestyle that will improve your asthma symptoms. These include:

■ giving up smoking (smoking can stop some types of preventer from working properly)
■ recognising and dealing with your personal asthma triggers
■ losing weight.

You should remain in regular contact with your GP or asthma nurse specialist and keep them informed of any changes in your symptoms. Remember, if your asthma interferes with your day-to-day way of living, it is not well controlled, and often a visit to your local surgery can put this right. There is good evidence that people undergoing regular checks have fewer asthma attacks, less time off work and enjoy a better quality of life.

LOSING WEIGHT MAY HELP TO IMPROVE YOUR ASTHMA SYMPTOMS.

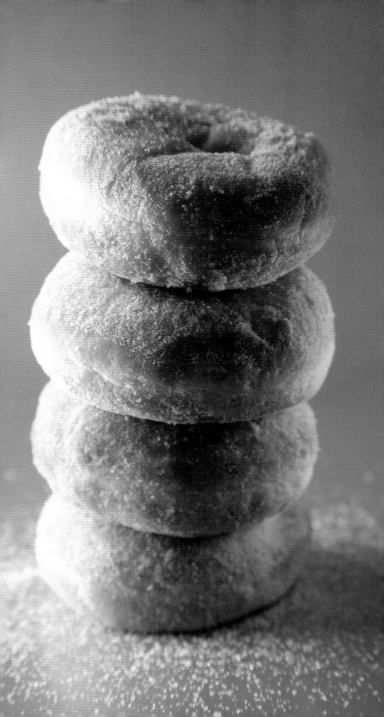

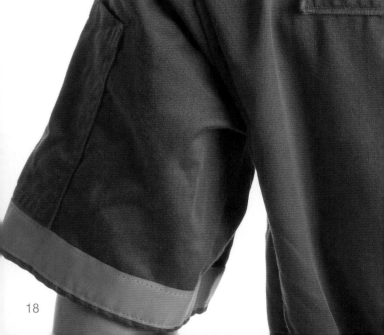

WHAT TO DO DURING AN ASTHMA ATTACK

1 Take your usual dose of reliever straight away.

2 Try to stay calm and to relax as much as your breathing will let you. Sit down, don't lie down, rest your hands on your knees to help support yourself and try to slow your breathing down as this will make you less exhausted.

3 Wait 5–10 minutes.

4 If the symptoms disappear, you should be able to go back to whatever you were doing.

5 If the reliever has no effect, call the doctor or 999.

6 Continue to take your reliever inhaler every few minutes until help arrives.

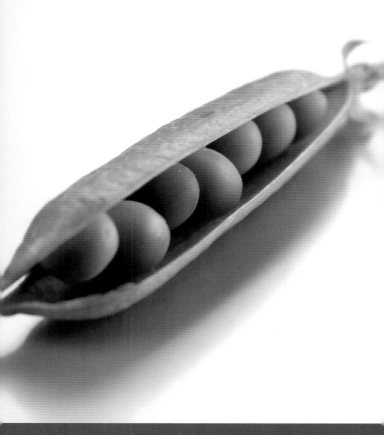

why me?

WHY ME?

If you, or a member of your family, has recently been diagnosed with asthma, you're not alone. Asthma is one of the most common chronic (long-term) diseases and affects between 100 and 150 million people worldwide.

Asthma can affect people of any age. Although many people develop asthma in childhood, asthma symptoms can appear at any time in life.

Over 5.2 million people in the UK are currently receiving treatment for asthma. That's 1.1 million children (1 in 10) and 4.1 million adults (1 in 12).

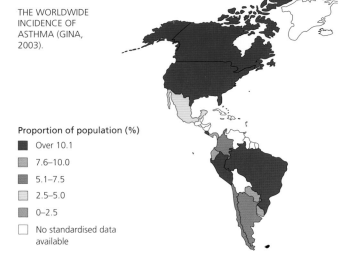

THE WORLDWIDE INCIDENCE OF ASTHMA (GINA, 2003).

Proportion of population (%)

- Over 10.1
- 7.6–10.0
- 5.1–7.5
- 2.5–5.0
- 0–2.5
- No standardised data available

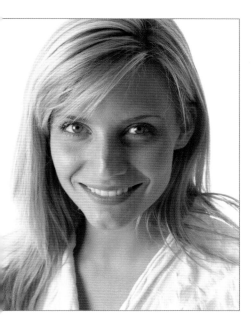

Asthma can be inherited – passed on from one family member to the next. A number of genetic (hereditary) and environmental factors influence the development of asthma. If one parent has asthma, the chance of their child developing asthma is roughly double that of children whose parents do not have asthma.

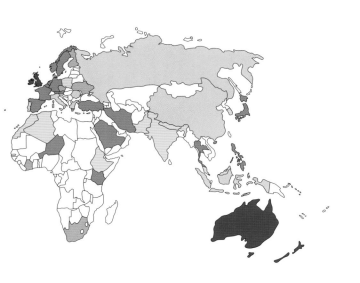

Although it is difficult to predict exactly who will get asthma, certain factors may make some people more likely to develop asthma than others. These include:

- ■ a family history of asthma or other allergy
- ■ smoking during pregnancy
- ■ exposure to irritants in the workplace.

Asthma tends to run in families that are prone to allergies. So, belonging to a family where some members have asthma and others have other allergies – such as eczema, hay fever (or allergic rhinitis) – can make you more likely to develop asthma.

Approximately 30–50% of the risk of developing asthma is caused by hereditary factors.

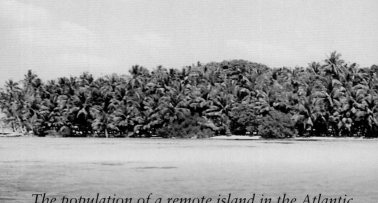

The population of a remote island in the Atlantic called Tristan da Cunha have provided many valuable clues regarding the inheritance of asthma.

There is no doubt that asthma is more common than it used to be. Currently, there is no definitive explanation for this. The increase in asthma has happened too quickly to be explained by genetic inheritance. What is more likely is that the substantial increase in asthma over recent years is linked to changes in our surrounding environment. Yet, whilst environmental air pollution generated by traffic, factories and power stations can make asthma symptoms worse, it has not been proven to actually cause asthma. Some scientists believe that it is far more likely that aspects of our indoor environment have influenced asthma development.

In Western Europe, the incidence of asthma has doubled in the last 10 years.

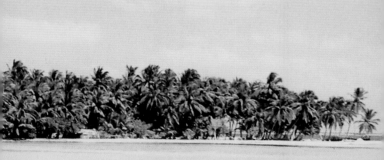

Following a shipwreck in 1892, 15 survivors settled on the island including 3 women with asthma. Following many years of breeding within a contained group of people, 1 in 3 of the islanders now has asthma.

WHY IS ASTHMA MORE COMMON THAN IT USED TO BE?

■ Asthma is diagnosed more often than it used to be. As a nation, we are more aware of our health and well-being and this may be helping to bring asthma into the public eye.

■ We are generally in better health than we used to be. Children who don't get many colds and other infections may have under-worked immune systems which may subsequently overreact to harmless things, such as pollen. This may cause asthma. This theory, which has been around since the 1990s, is known as the hygiene hypothesis.

■ Endotoxin is a poison produced by some types of bacteria that live in dusts, and can make asthma worse if it is inhaled. There is evidence to suggest that if we are exposed to endotoxin early on in life we may be protected against developing allergies. This may explain why children who grow up in rural settings and on farms, close to dusts and animals, are less likely to develop allergies and asthma.

■ Over recent years, our homes have become more energy efficient, which has meant less natural ventilation. As a result, fumes and gases generated within our homes are more likely to remain within the home, and may affect our airways.

- Our diet has changed. These days we eat more processed foods that contain artificial additives. These may exacerbate asthma.
- These days, we have a huge number of household cleaning products available to us. Substances such as bleach, paint stripper and carpet cleaner may be partly responsible for the recent rapid increase in asthma, although this is unconfirmed at the moment.

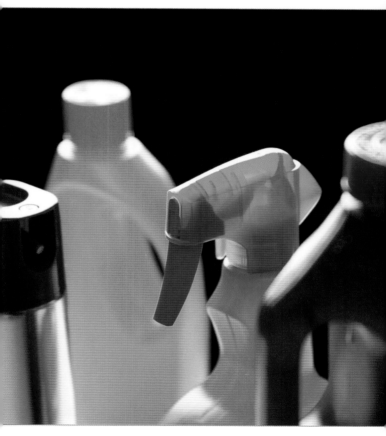

ASTHMA TRIGGERS

Asthma is an intermittent disease – it comes and goes – which means there may be times when your asthma is significantly worse. So what brings on an asthma attack? A number of different factors, or 'triggers', can contribute.

Asthma can be triggered by contact with something you are allergic to, cold weather, exercise or substances that irritate the airways. Common asthma triggers include:

- allergies (to):
  - house-dust mites
  - pollen
  - animal dander.
- irritants (cigarette smoke, chemical fumes)
- diet (food additives)
- certain types of medication (aspirin, beta-blockers)
- exercise.

Some 42% of people with asthma say that traffic fumes stop them from walking and shopping in congested areas.

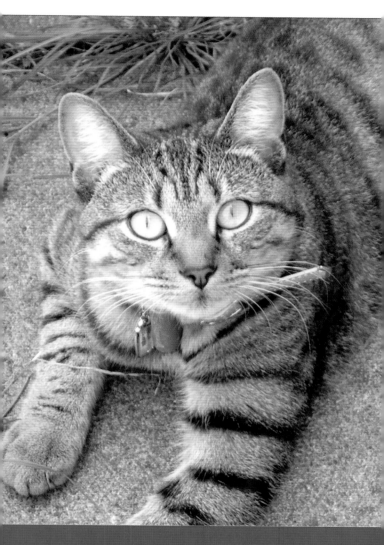

Avoiding asthma triggers is usually the best form of defence against all types of asthma.

THE HOUSE-DUST MITE

An allergy is a reaction that occurs when the immune system mistakenly identifies a normally harmless substance as damaging to the body.

The lowly house-dust mite can pose a serious threat to some people with asthma. Each night you could be sharing your bed with up to 1.5 million house-dust mites. Imagine that! The tiny creatures feed off scales of human skin and love warm, moist conditions. This makes your bed irresistible.

It is not the house-dust mites themselves, but their droppings (which are the size of grains of pollen), that worsen asthma and allergy in general. The droppings contain enzymes that the house-dust mite produces to break down hard-to-digest food, such as human skin scales. When people with a history of any kind of allergy are repeatedly exposed to house-dust mite droppings, they can develop a specific allergy to mites. Continued exposure to the dust mite allergens can then become a trigger for chronic symptoms.

An enzyme is a biological catalyst.

Dust mites live for between 3 and 4 months, and in this time, they produce up to 20 droppings a day. That's between 1,800 and 2,400 droppings per dust mite! If you consider that you have millions of dust mites living in your bed at any one time, this adds up to a lot of droppings.

PROFILE – HOUSE-DUST MITE

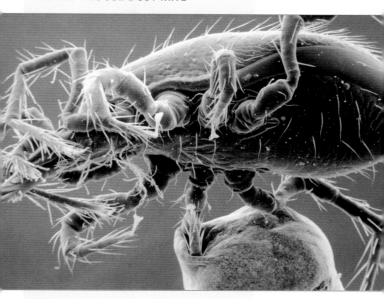

Name
Dermatophagoides pteronyssinus.

Size
Half the size of a full-stop.

Survives on
Moisture and oxygen from the atmosphere.

Likes
Human and animal skin scales, but will eat
pollen grains, insect scales, bacteria and
plant fibres.

Dislikes
Dry conditions.

Most dangerous weapon
Its droppings.

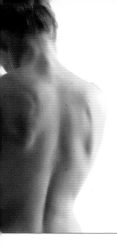

If you are sensitive, limiting the number of house-dust mites in your home may improve your asthma symptoms. The following steps may help (although definitive scientific evidence is lacking).

1. Vacuum throughout your home on a regular basis.
2. Hot wash (at 60°C) sheets, duvet covers and pillowcases.
3. Freeze soft toys for at least 6 hours on a regular basis.
4. Use specially designed bed-coverings on your mattress, duvet and pillows. These coverings may improve your asthma symptoms by forming a barrier between you and the dust mites in your bed.

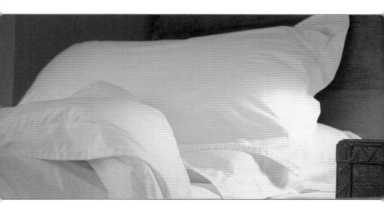

ASTHMA AND SMOKING

Smoking kills 120,000 people in the UK every year and is the single most preventable cause of early death in the world (Cancer Research UK). Cigarette smoke damages the airways of the lung and can cause potentially life-threatening diseases such as chronic obstructive pulmonary disease (COPD).

For people with asthma, smoking is a real problem. Cigarette smoke can damage the lungs and may stop certain asthma drugs, like inhaled corticosteroids (a type of preventer), from working properly. Even in people who do not smoke, inhaling second-hand cigarette smoke can make symptoms worse and can even trigger an asthma attack.

Despite the considerable evidence that smoking can make asthma more difficult to manage, approximately 25% of adults with asthma continue to smoke. If you smoke and have asthma, or you live with someone who has asthma, it is important that you try to give up. Many doctors, hospitals and local health authorities run support groups and courses to help. Your healthcare team can tell you what facilities are available in your area.

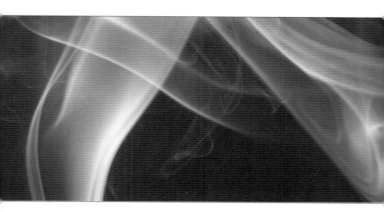

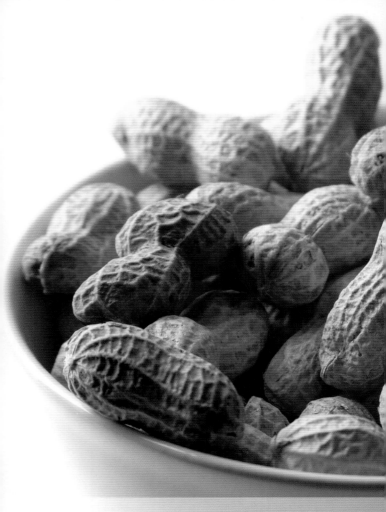

ASTHMA AND FOOD

Although food-triggered asthma is unusual, certain foods or food additives may bring about an asthma attack in some people. Food additives are substances added to food to preserve its quality, texture, taste or colour. The UK Food Standards Agency has identified a number of food additives that may affect the airways and worsen asthma.

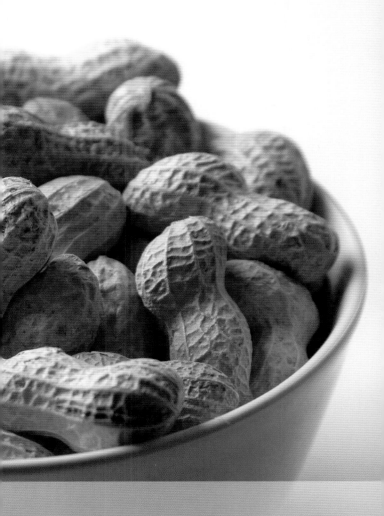

Identifying exactly which foods worsen asthma has been the focus of much scientific investigation. Food allergens have been found in milk, eggs, peanuts, tree nuts, wheat, fish and shellfish. However, it is important to emphasise that these foods will only trigger asthma in a very small number of susceptible people.

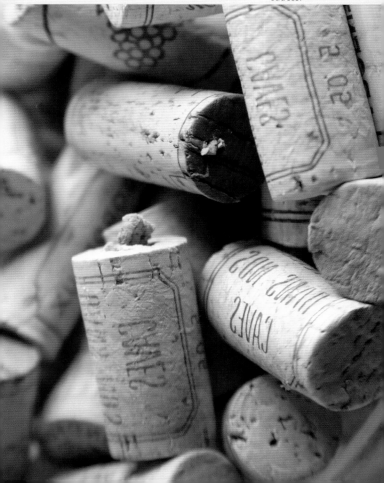

FOOD ADDITIVES THAT MAY AFFECT THE AIRWAYS AND WORSEN ASTHMA

Additive	E-number	What is it used for?	Where is it found?
Sulphur dioxide and other sulphites	E220, E221, E222, E223, E224, E226, E227	To preserve food	Soft drinks, sausages, burgers, dried fruit, vegetables, wine, beer, pickled foods.
Benzoic acid and other benzoates	E210, E211, E212, E213, E214, E215, E216, E217	To preserve food	Soft drinks, fruit, honey.
Tartrazine	E102	To colour food	Soft drinks, sweets, sauces.

IS ALL ASTHMA THE SAME?

Although the basic symptoms of asthma are
very similar from one person to the next, the
circumstances under which asthma attacks can
be brought on may vary considerably. The
different types of asthma include:

- occupational asthma
- aspirin-sensitive asthma
- exercise-induced asthma.

Occupational asthma

Occupational asthma is asthma that is
triggered by a substance that is unique to your
working environment. Occupational asthma
can take weeks, months or even years to
develop, depending on the person and the
substance involved. Occupational asthma can
occur in:

- smokers and non-smokers
- people who have had asthma before and
  those who have not
- people who have recently changed jobs
  and people who have been in the same job
  for many years.

COMMON CAUSES OF OCCUPATIONAL ASTHMA

Cause of occupational asthma	Who is most at risk?
Animals (e.g. animal urine, grain mites, moths)	Animal handlers, laboratory workers, farmers, grain-store workers.
Plants (e.g. grain dust, flour of wheat or rye, latex)	Grain-store workers, bakers, millers, laboratory workers, healthcare professionals.
Enzymes	Detergent industry workers, laboratory workers, bakers.
Wood dusts or barks	Builders, carpenters.
Drugs	Laboratory workers, healthcare workers.
Metals	Workers in the steel industry.

So who is most at risk of developing occupational asthma? Some of the major causes are outlined in the table above.

You can identify occupational asthma by asking yourself a number of simple questions.

- Are your symptoms better on days away from work?
- Are your symptoms better when you are on holiday?
- Did you first notice your symptoms fairly soon after starting a new job?
- Did you first notice your symptoms shortly after you changed your work conditions within the same job?

If you think you may have developed occupational asthma, you should seek medical advice straight away. As well as your GP, occupational therapists – health professionals who are trained to help people regain the ability to perform their activities of daily living – will also be able to help. To assist your doctor in

There are up to 3,000 new cases of occupational asthma reported in the UK each year.

making a diagnosis, you can keep a record of when your symptoms occur. Your GP may also organise certain laboratory tests, in which you are exposed to low levels of the suspected workplace allergen under controlled conditions. If the substance triggers your symptoms, then it is likely you have developed an allergy to it. Occupational rhinitis – worked-related sneezing, or a runny or blocked nose – often develops into occupational asthma.

Once occupational asthma has been diagnosed, ideally, you should change your working conditions. This may mean transferring elsewhere within your company, or retraining completely. If you remove yourself from the cause of your asthma at an early stage, you can usually 'turn it off'. However, if you leave it too late, it won't go away. It is your employer's legal responsibility to accommodate your needs and you should not suffer discrimination as a result of your condition. You may even be eligible for some kind of workers' compensation. For more advice on occupational asthma, contact your local Health and Safety Executive (HSE) office *(www.hse.gov.uk).*

Around 10% of all cases of adult asthma can be related to allergen exposure in the workplace.

Occupational asthma is usually diagnosed by taking five lung function measurements on three separate occasions. One when you are at work, one when you are off work, and one when you are away from work on holiday.

Aspirin-sensitive asthma

For the vast majority of people, taking aspirin for headaches or other common medical ailments does not affect their asthma. However, for a very small proportion of people with asthma (perhaps 3–5%), aspirin, along with similar, so-called non-steroidal anti-inflammatory drugs (NSAIDs; e.g. ibuprofen), can cause asthma to worsen, often provoking a severe and sudden attack. Read the labels and package inserts of pain-relieving drugs carefully before you use them. Check the small print. Many of these will carry a warning to people with asthma.

Aspirin was introduced onto the drug market in 1899, and within a few years, it had become one of the most popular drugs on Earth.

COMMONLY USED MEDICATIONS THAT CONTAIN ASPIRIN AND MAY WORSEN ASTHMA	
Brand name	Active ingredients
Alka-Seltzer®	aspirin
Anadin®	aspirin, caffeine
Anadin Extra Soluble®	aspirin, caffeine, paracetamol
Angettes 75®	aspirin
Askit®	aspirin, caffeine
Aspro Clear®	aspirin
Beechams Lemon Tablets®	aspirin
Beechams Powders®	aspirin, caffeine
Caprin®	aspirin
Codis 500®	aspirin, codeine
Disprin®	aspirin
Disprin Extra®	aspirin, paracetamol
Phensic®	aspirin, caffeine

Why does aspirin do this? People with asthma who are sensitive to aspirin produce excessive quantities of natural chemicals called leukotrienes. At the moment it remains a mystery exactly why this is, but it may all be linked to the way in which aspirin works in the body – its mechanism of action. Leukotrienes cause the muscles surrounding the bronchial tubes to contract, narrowing the airways and causing the person to wheeze and lose their breath.

Some of the newer drugs used to treat asthma work by preventing leukotrienes from doing what they normally do, and are called leukotriene receptor antagonists. Montelukast (Singulair®) is an example of one such drug.

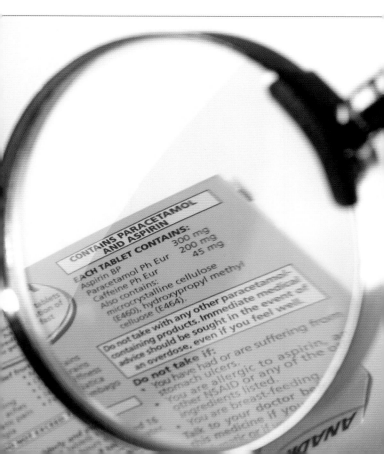

Exercise-induced asthma

In the UK, about 21% of people with asthma (1.1 million) experience severe breathing problems whilst they are jogging or running.

For some people, certain types of exercise can trap air in the airways and make it difficult to breathe. Sometimes, exercise can even bring on an asthma attack. Some evidence suggests that 'exercise-induced' asthma is due to the increased cooling and drying of the airways that occurs when we breathe faster and deeper, during or after exercise. Some types of exercise will cause more wheeziness or chest tightness than others. For example, running outside is generally worse than swimming.

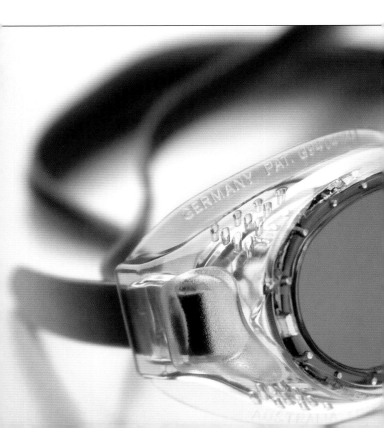

It may seem ironic, but in general, exercise is very good for asthma. People with well-controlled asthma should be able to take part in almost any type of sport. Those people with very severe asthma may find their options more limited and should discuss them with their healthcare professional. If you find that your asthma is beginning to restrict your exercise when it did not in the past, it is important that you consult your GP. It may be a sign your asthma is getting worse.

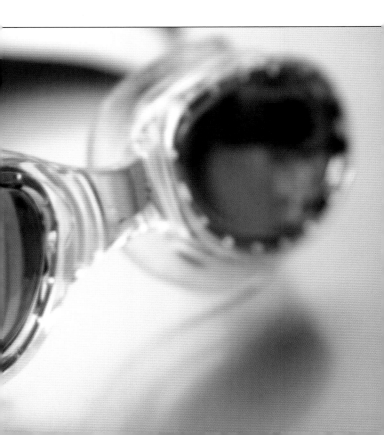

Asthma, exercise and school

It is important that children with asthma (with the exception of those children with severe asthma) participate in the full curriculum of sports and physical education offered in their school. Exercising regularly is extremely beneficial to our general health and may stop your child developing type 2 diabetes or heart disease in later life, conditions which are strongly associated with being overweight and inactive.

Children with well-controlled asthma will be able to enjoy sport at school without worrying about their asthma. Since there is a chance that some children may experience symptoms during sports lessons, it is important that teachers and supervisors are aware of this. However, you should bear in mind that teaching staff are under no legal obligation to administer asthma medication to your child. It is your, and to some extent your child's, responsibility to make sure their asthma medication is available to them should they need it.

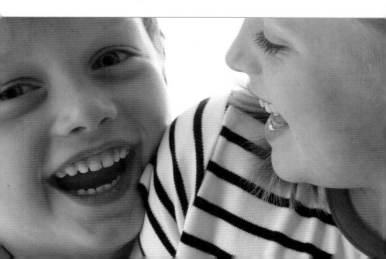

ASTHMA THROUGH HISTORY

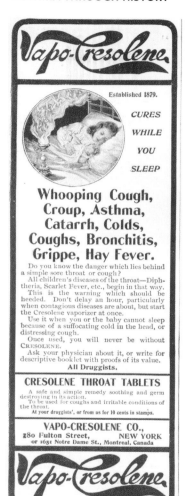

COURTESY OF MARK SANDERS,
www.inhalatorium.com

■ Asthma-like symptoms were first recorded over 3,500 years ago in an Egyptian manuscript.

■ The Greek philosopher, Hippocrates, was the first to coin the term, 'asthma', which means 'laboured breathing' in Greek.

■ Records, dating back as far as 1,500 BC, indicate that asthma was considered to be a disease caused by 'spirits'.

■ It was during the seventeenth and eighteenth centuries that physicians first realised asthma was caused by constrictions of the airways.

■ In 1678, the physician, Thomas Willis, described asthma as the 'obstruction of bronchi by thick humors, swelling of their walls and obstruction from without'.

■ Sir John Floyer first suggested that asthma was due to spasms of bronchial smooth muscle in 1698.

■ Not until the 1970s did it become clear that asthma was a chronic inflammatory disorder of the airways.

■ Famous people to have suffered from asthma include Ludwig Van Beethoven, Charles Dickens and John F Kennedy.

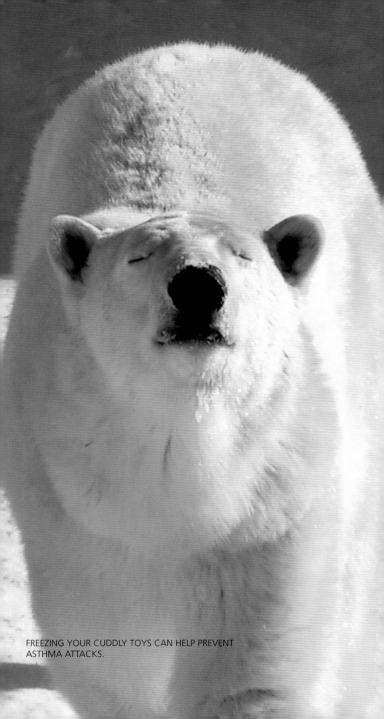

FREEZING YOUR CUDDLY TOYS CAN HELP PREVENT ASTHMA ATTACKS.

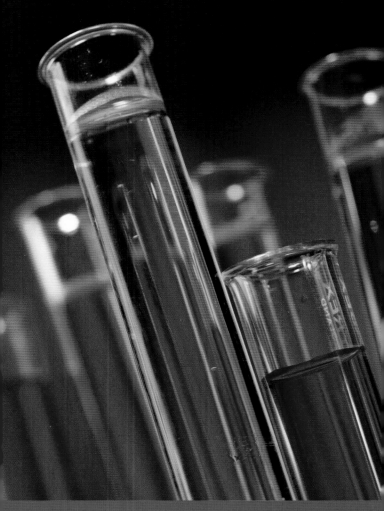

simple science

SIMPLE SCIENCE

Asthma is closely tied in with the processes of inflammation and smooth muscle contraction.

INFLAMMATION

Inflammatory cells are tiny, mobile structures that flock to and accumulate in inflamed areas of the body. Mast cells, eosinophils and neutrophils are all inflammatory cells.

Inflammatory mediators are chemicals made by the body that control the process of inflammation. Histamine, cytokines and leukotrienes are all inflammatory mediators.

Inflammation is the body's way of responding to injury, infection or invasion by foreign bodies. In the case of asthma, the foreign bodies that cause inflammation may be pollen grains, animal fur, house-dust mites or air pollutants. It depends on the individual person.

In asthma, our immune system attacks these foreign bodies by sending white blood cells to the scene. These so-called 'inflammatory cells' release histamine, cytokines and leukotrienes – chemicals made by our bodies that perpetuate the inflammation process. As a result, our airways become red, inflamed and produce mucus in an attempt to get rid of the foreign invaders. In people with asthma the smooth muscle that lines the airways is hypersensitive and tightens up. This combination of events means that breathing in and out becomes difficult. Inflammation is closely linked to allergy although you can have asthma without having other allergies and vice versa.

simple science

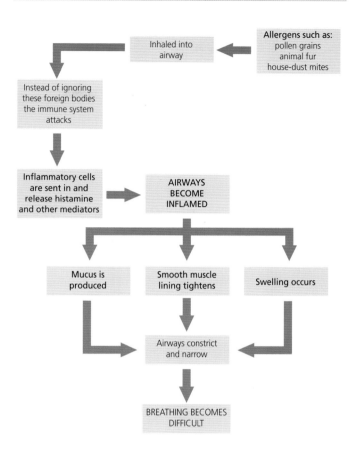

IN ASTHMA

■ The airways become over-sensitive to irritating substances.
This may be due to allergy.

■ The airways produce too much mucus which may plug them
up in places.

47

Cell	Pronunciation	What does it do?
Eosinophil	Ee-o-sihn-o-fil	Fights foreign invaders and participates in allergic reactions.
Macrophage	Mac-crow-pharge	Name means 'big eater'. Helps to protect the body by 'eating-up' damaged or foreign invaders. Releases cytokines.
Mast cell	–	Makes and releases histamine and other inflammatory mediators. Causes inflammation during allergic reactions.
Neutrophil	Noo-tro-fil	Helps to protect the body by 'eating-up' damaged or foreign cells. The first to arrive on the scene.
T lymphocyte	T-limp-foe-sight	Part of the immune system. Attacks foreign invaders.

Mediator	Pronunciation	What does it do?
Histamine	Hiss-tar-mean	Released during an allergic reaction. Causes swelling, heat, redness and itching.
Prostaglandins	–	Powerful in small quantities. Mediates a number of inflammatory responses.
Leukotrienes	Lew-ko-try-eens	Powerful in small quantities. Mediates a number of inflammatory responses.
Cytokines	Sigh-tow-kines	Large group of chemicals (more than 100). Carry messages that promote inflammation.

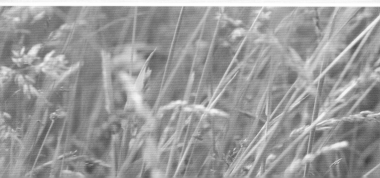

MUSCLE CONTRACTION

The bronchi in our lungs are made up of rings of smooth muscle. Normally, this smooth muscle is relaxed, our airways are open and breathing is easy. The smooth muscle is maintained in this relaxed state by a complex process that amongst other things involves adrenaline. Adrenaline is always present in our bloodstream and is vitally important for a number of reasons:

Smooth muscle is usually found in the walls of hollow organs and works automatically without you being aware of it.

■ it quickens our heart rate
■ it quickens our pulse
■ it keeps our airways open.

Adrenaline (and a similar substance called noradrenaline) binds to structures called β_2-adrenoceptors on the surface of airway smooth muscle. This keeps the muscle relaxed, the airways open and helps us to breathe easily.

In asthma, this natural balance is upset. The muscle in the airways contracts, the airway opening is narrowed and breathing becomes much more of an effort.

Adrenaline is responsible for the 'fight or flight' reaction that helps us respond to threatening situations (like coming face-to-face with a bull whilst crossing a field!).

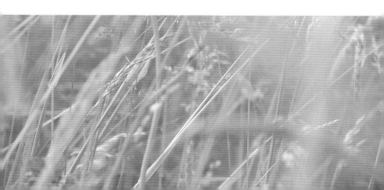

Relaxed

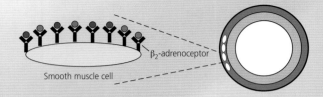

β₂-adrenoceptor

Smooth muscle cell

Contracted

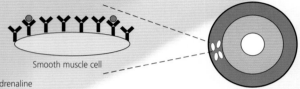

Smooth muscle cell

● Noradrenaline
● β₂-agonist

BRONCHODILATORS
WORK BY
MIMICKING
THE RELAXING
EFFECTS OF
NORADRENALINE.

HOW DO ASTHMA DRUGS WORK?

Bronchodilators

Bronchodilators are drugs that open (or
dilate) the airways by mimicking the action
of noradrenaline. They occupy the same
β_2-adrenoceptors that noradrenaline would
otherwise occupy on the surface of smooth
muscle cells and trigger the same effect. This
means they help to relax smooth muscle.
For this reason they are also known as
β_2-agonists. An agonist is a drug that binds
to a receptor and produces the same
biological effect as the naturally occurring
substance. An antagonist therefore is a drug
that blocks the effect of a naturally occurring
substance like noradrenaline.

Salbutamol (Ventolin®), terbutaline
(Bricanyl®), salmeterol (Serevent®) and
formoterol (Foradil®, Oxis®) are β_2-agonists.

Anti-inflammatory drugs

As their name suggests, anti-inflammatory drugs reverse the inflammation that occurs in the airways in asthma. By attacking the inflammatory cells and their inflammatory mediators, these drugs reduce the swelling and redness of the airways and stop the production of the clogging mucus. They also help to calm down irritation of the airways.

These drugs can take a while to get going, but once they get inside inflammatory cells, they stop them from making their inflammatory mediators and reduce inflammation. Corticosteroids (different from the anabolic steroids that some bodybuilders might use), are the main type of anti-inflammatory drug used to control inflammation in asthma.

Corticosteroids can be inhaled, or given as tablets in certain circumstances, to bring severe inflammation under control quickly and to settle down a flare-up (known as an exacerbation) of asthma.

Inhaled corticosteroids such as beclometasone (Becotide®) and budesonide (Pulmicort®) have become established worldwide as the cornerstones of preventer medication in asthma.

A new class of anti-inflammatory drug (montelukast [Singulair®]) has recently been introduced that is not a corticosteroid and which is available as a tablet. It works by blocking the inflammatory mediator leukotriene which is why it is known as a 'leukotriene receptor antagonist'.

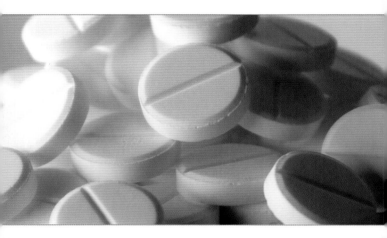

A detailed scientific review of the available evidence on the drugs used to manage asthma can be found in BESTMEDICINE Asthma, *available from www.bestmedicine.com*

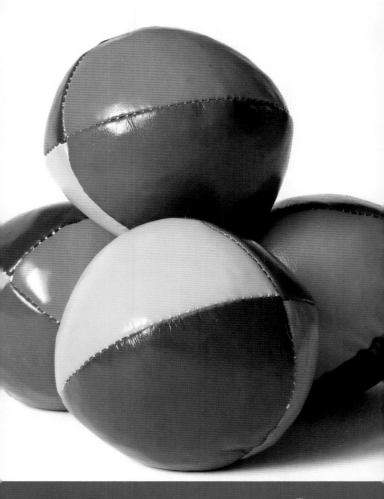

managing
asthma

MANAGING ASTHMA

The key to effective asthma control lies in an effective asthma management programme.

HOW WILL ASTHMA AFFECT MY LIFE?

If you have recently been diagnosed with asthma then it's only natural that you will worry about how it will affect your life. Of course, if you have been living with asthma for many years then you will be well aware of what living with asthma means, although you may be unaware of certain, simple preventative measures you can take to improve matters.

Millions of people with asthma continue to lead normal lives. So there's no reason why you can't take control of your symptoms and lead a full and active life. Of course, in order to do this, you will need some help, and your local health authority has vast experience in looking after people with asthma. There are also a number of asthma support groups, both locally and nationally. Asthma UK is an independent organisation that provides the latest advice and information to people with asthma (*www.asthma.org.uk*).

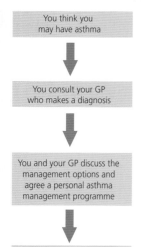

You think you may have asthma

You consult your GP who makes a diagnosis

You and your GP discuss the management options and agree a personal asthma management programme

Your asthma is controlled

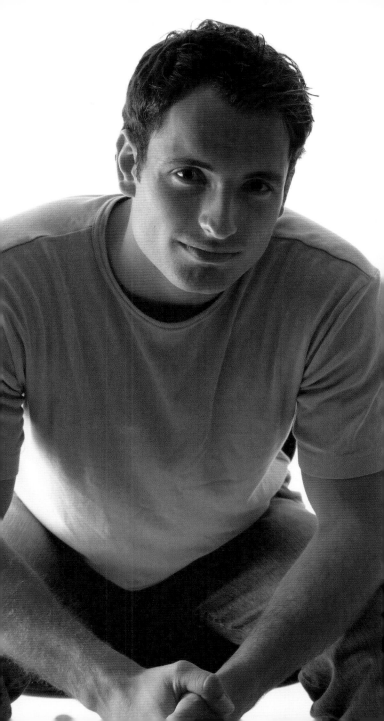

DIAGNOSIS

Asthma is usually diagnosed on the basis of a number of 'lung function' tests (which monitor how well your lungs are working) and the symptoms you describe to your GP.

Your doctor will ask you a number of questions about your symptoms and listen to your chest to find out how well your airways are working. Putting your symptoms into words can be difficult. It may help to think about how you would answer the following questions before you get into the consultation room.

Peak expiratory flow (PEF) is a measure of how fast you can breathe out.

- How does it feel when you have breathing problems?
- Do you cough or wheeze? Does your chest feel tight?
- How long have you been having problems?
- At what time of the day do your symptoms occur?
- Have you had difficulty sleeping because of your symptoms?
- Is there anything in particular that seems to set off your symptoms?
- Did you or anyone in your family have asthma, eczema or hay fever when you/they were a child?
- Are you taking aspirin, ibuprofen or a beta-blocker? If so, do they make your symptoms worse?
- Do you smoke yourself or breathe in second-hand smoke?

Your GP will use an instrument called a peak flow meter to measure your peak expiratory flow (PEF) – how fast you can blow out air after taking a deep breath. Your peak flow gives valuable clues about the severity of your asthma. When asthma is well controlled, there should be very little difference between peak flow readings from one day to the next. It is important that people with asthma learn how to measure their peak flow and make a note of it on a regular basis. Many people with asthma keep a 'peak flow diary' and report back to their GP at regular scheduled visits. The peak flow meter is easy to use, your doctor will show you how, and it is available on prescription from the NHS and from your local pharmacist.

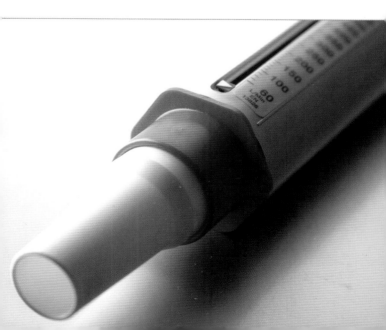

WHAT IS A NORMAL PEAK FLOW?

Peak flow readings vary according to your age, size and sex. The actual value itself is not as important as the way in which your peak flow readings may vary from day to day. If you have asthma, your peak flow will vary before and after exercise, or before and after you are exposed to one of your asthma triggers. Even in healthy people, peak flow readings vary slightly from time to time. The reading is often slightly higher in the evening compared with the morning.

If you are given a peak flow meter, it is important that you know how to use it properly, so that the measurements you take are accurate. The following guidance will help.

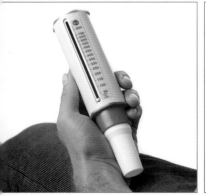

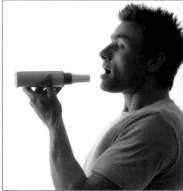

1. Check that the pointer is at zero.

2. Stand or sit in a comfortable, upright position.

3. Hold the peak flow meter level (horizontally) and keep your fingers away from the pointer.

4. Take a deep breath and close your lips firmly around the mouthpiece.

5. Blow as hard as you can.

6. Look at the pointer and check your reading.

7. Reset the pointer back to zero.

8. Repeat three times and record the highest reading in your asthma diary.

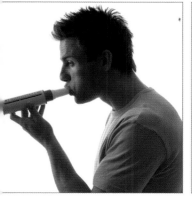

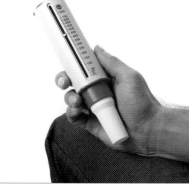

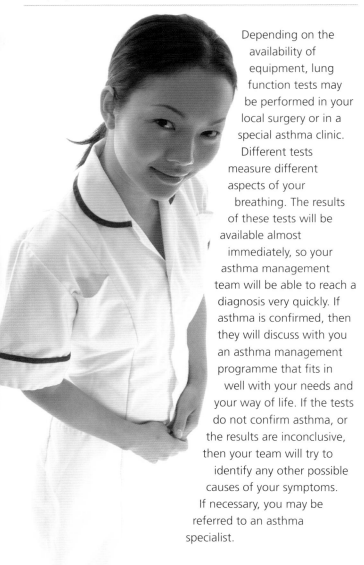

Depending on the availability of equipment, lung function tests may be performed in your local surgery or in a special asthma clinic. Different tests measure different aspects of your breathing. The results of these tests will be available almost immediately, so your asthma management team will be able to reach a diagnosis very quickly. If asthma is confirmed, then they will discuss with you an asthma management programme that fits in well with your needs and your way of life. If the tests do not confirm asthma, or the results are inconclusive, then your team will try to identify any other possible causes of your symptoms. If necessary, you may be referred to an asthma specialist.

TESTING LUNG FUNCTION

Lung function tests measure different aspects of your breathing.

Peak expiratory flow (PEF) (Usually referred to as 'peak flow')

Measures the fastest rate of air flow as you expel air when breathing out.
Peak flow can be easily measured at home and can be used to monitor when
you may need to change your medication or seek medical help. You may be
asked to record your results in a peak flow diary.

Spirometry

Spirometric tests are performed in a doctor's surgery or hospital clinic. You
will be asked to breathe in and out through a mouthpiece whilst a machine
measures your air flow. These tests record:

- vital capacity (VC) – the maximum volume of air you can breathe in or out
- forced expiratory volume in 1 second (FEV_1) – the volume of air you
  breathe out in the first second after a maximal inspiration. Measures how
  quickly full lungs can be emptied.

Bronchial provocation test

In asthma, the airways may narrow in response to certain irritating
substances. Metacholine and histamine are irritating substances that can be
safely administered under controlled conditions.

The provocation test measures how much narrowing occurs after you inhale
small amounts of sprays containing histamine or metacholine. You may be
required to inhale between 5 and 8 different strengths of spray (starting with
the weakest strength) during the test. Spirometry measurements (see above)
are taken shortly after each inhalation.

Exercise tests

Exercise-induced asthma is a condition in which the airways narrow
significantly during vigorous exercise. During tests for exercise-induced
asthma, spirometric readings are taken before and after running on a
treadmill or riding an exercise bicycle.

SOUNDS LIKE ASTHMA, LOOKS LIKE ASTHMA, BUT COULD IT BE SOMETHING ELSE?

Asthma shares a number of symptoms with other respiratory disorders, including chronic obstructive pulmonary disease (COPD), bronchiectasis, cystic fibrosis and bronchiolitis. Your GP may need to rule some of these out before asthma can be diagnosed. A number of important clues can alert your doctor to asthma, including:

- variation in the severity of symptoms
- coming and going of symptoms
- worsening of symptoms at night
- worsening of symptoms by recognised triggers.

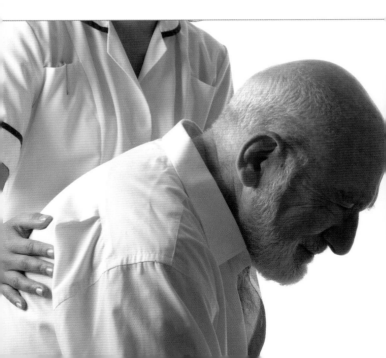

RESPIRATORY DISORDERS THAT SHARE SOME SYMPTOMS WITH ASTHMA

Disease	Definition
Asthma	A reversible inflammatory lung disease characterised by tightened and narrowed airways.
Bronchiolitis	Inflammation of the bronchioles, the smallest branches of the respiratory system, as a result of a viral infection. Bronchiolitis mostly affects infants and young children, and can cause wheezing and serious difficulty in breathing.
Chronic obstructive pulmonary disease (COPD)	A term used to describe two lung diseases – emphysema and chronic bronchitis. *Emphysema* The lungs produce too much mucus, and the alveoli become damaged. It becomes difficult to breathe and to get enough oxygen into the blood. The main cause of emphysema is long-term smoking. *Chronic bronchitis* The membranes lining the larger bronchial tubes become inflamed, and an excessive amount of mucus is produced. The person develops a bad cough to get rid of the mucus.
Common cold	The most common respiratory infection. Symptoms may include a mild temperature, cough, headache, runny nose, sneezing and sore throat.
Cystic fibrosis (CF)	The most common inherited (genetic) disease affecting the lungs. The mucus produced by the body is abnormally thick and sticky and can clog the airways and make a person more vulnerable to bacterial infections.
Lung cancer	Caused by an abnormal growth of cells in the lungs, the most common cause of lung cancer is smoking. Usually starts in the lining of the bronchi, and takes a long time to develop. Symptoms include a persistent cough that may bring up blood, chest pain, hoarseness, a shortness of breath and weight loss.
Pneumonia	An inflammation of the lungs that usually occurs following a bacterial or viral infection. Pneumonia causes fever and inflammation of lung tissue, and makes breathing difficult.

DIAGNOSING ASTHMA IN CHILDREN

Diagnosing asthma in small children or infants is considerably more difficult than diagnosing asthma in adults. This is mainly because children are unable to put into words exactly how they feel and under what circumstances their symptoms get better or worse. Your GP will rely on you to describe your child's symptoms accurately.

Unfortunately, the key diagnostic test – the peak flow meter – does not work particularly well in children under the age of 6, although low-range models have been specially designed for young children. Your GP may request that you keep a diary of your child's symptoms and may ask you about the following in order to decide whether or not your child has asthma:

- a family history of asthma or hay fever
- signs of allergies to pollen, animals or exercise
- a recent viral infection
- whether you smoke around your child or smoked during your pregnancy
- whether your child was born prematurely.

Children whose parents smoke are 1.5 times more likely to develop asthma.

GUIDELINES USED TO CLASSIFY ASTHMA SEVERITY (GINA).

	Asthma severity	Lung function	
		PEF or FEV$_1$	PEF variability
	Severe	60%	>30%
Persistent	Moderate	>60–80%	>30%
	Mild	80%	20–30%
Intermittent	Mild	80%	<20%

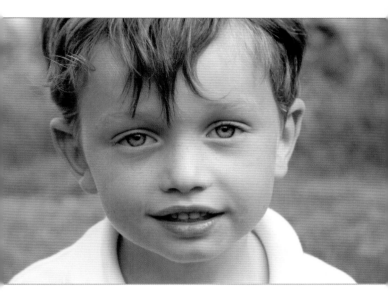

HOW BAD IS YOUR ASTHMA?

Your GP will rate the severity of your asthma
according to:

- how much it interferes with your day-to-
  day lifestyle
- the intensity and frequency of your
  symptoms
- how much your lung function changes
  from one day to the next
- the type and dose of asthma medication
  that is required to control your asthma.

Symptom frequency	Nocturnal symptoms	Exacerbations
Continual	Frequent	Frequent
Daily	>1/week	Affect activity
>2/week<1/day	>2/month	May affect activity
2/week	2/month	Are brief

ASTHMA MANAGEMENT PROGRAMME

Once a diagnosis of asthma has been confirmed, your GP (and other members of your asthma management team) will put together a personal asthma management plan to help you to control your asthma. If you have any questions regarding any aspect of your asthma, it is important to ask a member of your management team. They will be happy to help.

Any asthma treatment programme should aim to:

- reduce your asthma symptoms
- limit the amount of medication you have to take
- reduce your emergency visits to hospital
- improve your quality of life.

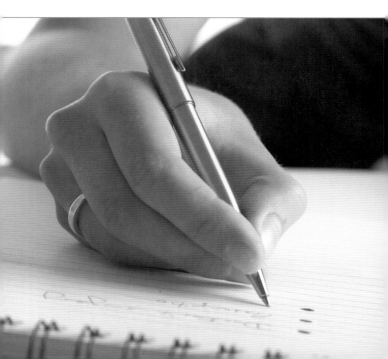

WHAT TO DO DURING AN ASTHMA ATTACK

1. Take your usual dose of reliever straight away.

2. Try to stay calm and to relax as much as your breathing will let you. Sit down, don't lie down, rest your hands on your knees to help support yourself and try to slow your breathing down as this will make you less exhausted.

3. Wait 5–10 minutes.

4. If the symptoms disappear, you should be able to go back to whatever you were doing.

5. If the reliever has no effect, call a doctor or an ambulance.

6. Continue to take your reliever inhaler every few minutes until help arrives.

Rarely, you may experience a severe or perhaps even life-threatening episode of asthma that does not respond to your normal asthma medications. This must be treated in hospital. You may be given the following:

- high-flow oxygen via a mask
- normal asthma medications via a nebuliser
- high doses of corticosteroids as tablets.

You may be kept in hospital until your peak flow has returned to normal and your asthma symptoms have been controlled.

LIFESTYLE CHANGES

In the first instance, your asthma management team may recommend some changes you can make to your lifestyle that will immediately improve your asthma symptoms. These include:

- recognising and dealing with your personal asthma triggers (e.g. animals, tobacco smoke, house-dust mites)
- changing your diet
- losing weight
- stopping smoking.

Whilst adopting some of these measures may make your asthma easier to deal with, it is important that you don't let asthma take over your life.

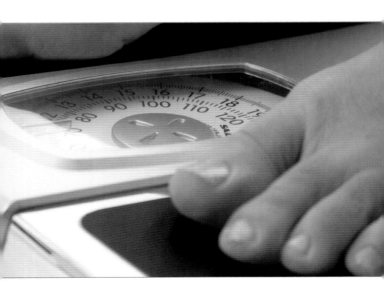

Pets

Animals can often trigger asthma symptoms. Up to 56% of people with asthma are sensitive to pet allergens. Aggravating allergens can be found in your pet's dead skin flakes (dander), urine, saliva and fur. Exposure to these substances can worsen your symptoms and trigger an acute asthma attack. The most effective way of controlling animal allergens is not to allow animals in the home. If pets are one of your asthma triggers, you should seriously consider finding them a new home. If this is too drastic a measure, it is important that you limit the areas in the home in which pets are allowed to wander. You should try to keep pets:

- out of sleeping areas and bedrooms
- away from upholstered furniture and carpets
- away from stuffed toys
- outside (as much as possible).

It is also important to keep your pet clean and well groomed, provided that all grooming is done by a non-asthmatic member of the household. Vacuuming carpets, rugs and furniture at least twice a week and washing bedclothes at a temperature of at least 60°C, will also help to reduce levels of animal allergens in the home.

THE DRUG TREATMENT OF ASTHMA

In addition to recommending that you change certain elements of your lifestyle, your asthma management team will also discuss with you the best course of drug treatment to suit your needs. The overriding purpose of any drug treatment strategy is to control your asthma symptoms, improve your lung function and prevent asthma attacks.

Asthma treatments can be separated into two main types – preventers and relievers. If taken according to your doctor's recommendations and used regularly, preventers will help to stop asthma attacks from occurring in the first place. Although relievers will help you to control your asthma symptoms in the event of an attack, they do not affect the root of the problem (the inflammation) and are therefore more of a temporary control measure. Sometimes, preventers and relievers can be given together.

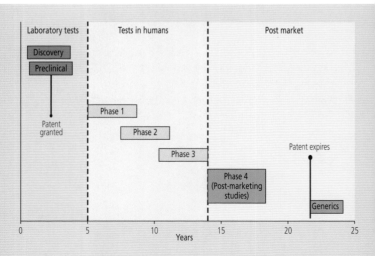

THE DRUG DEVELOPMENT PROCESS

Developing and launching a new drug onto the commercial market is an extremely costly and time-consuming venture. The process can take a pharmaceutical company between 10 and 15 years from the outset, at an estimated cost of £500 million. Much of this time is spent fulfilling strict guidelines set out by regulatory authorities in order to ensure the safety and quality of the end product. Once registered, a new drug is protected by a patent for 20 years, after which time other rival companies are free to manufacture and market identical drugs, called generics. Thus, the pharmaceutical company has a finite period of time before patent expiry to recoup the costs of drug development and return a profit to their shareholders.

During the development process, a drug undergoes five distinct phases of rigorous testing – the preclinical phase, which takes place in the laboratory – and phases 1, 2, 3 and 4, which involve testing in humans. Approval from the regulatory body and hence, a licence to sell the drug, is dependent on the satisfactory completion of all phases of testing. In the UK, the Medicines and Healthcare Products Regulatory Agency (MHRA) and the European Medicines Evaluation Agency (EMEA) regulate the drug development process.

- Only about 1 in every 100 drugs that enter the preclinical stage progress into human testing because they failed to work or had unacceptable side-effects.
- Animal testing is an important part of drug development. Before a drug reaches a human, it is vital that its basic safety has been established in an animal. Researchers do everything in their powers to minimise the number of animals they use and must adhere to strict guidelines issued by the Home Office.
- Phase 1 testing takes place in groups of 10–80 healthy volunteers.
- Phase 2 testing takes place in 100–300 patients diagnosed with the disease the drug is designed to treat.
- Phase 3 clinical trials involve between 1,000 and 3,000 patients with the relevant disease, and look at both the short- and long-term effects of the drug.
- Phase 4 testing and monitoring continues after the drug has reached the market.

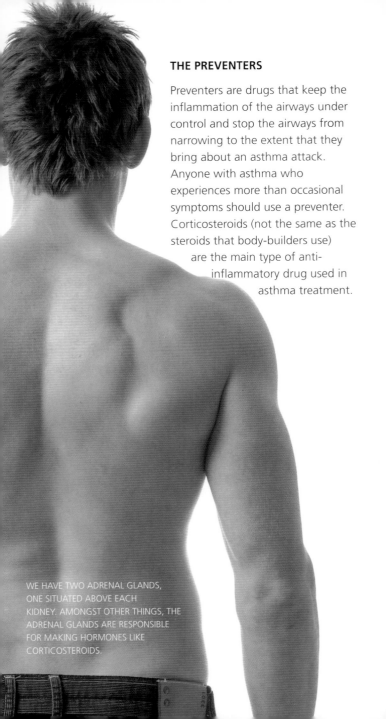

THE PREVENTERS

Preventers are drugs that keep the inflammation of the airways under control and stop the airways from narrowing to the extent that they bring about an asthma attack. Anyone with asthma who experiences more than occasional symptoms should use a preventer. Corticosteroids (not the same as the steroids that body-builders use) are the main type of anti-inflammatory drug used in asthma treatment.

WE HAVE TWO ADRENAL GLANDS, ONE SITUATED ABOVE EACH KIDNEY. AMONGST OTHER THINGS, THE ADRENAL GLANDS ARE RESPONSIBLE FOR MAKING HORMONES LIKE CORTICOSTEROIDS.

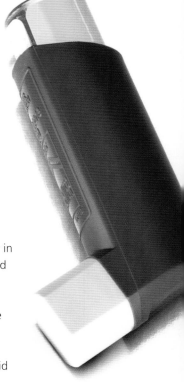

Inhaled corticosteroids

Corticosteroids are made naturally in the body by the adrenal glands and help to reduce inflammation. In addition to their role in asthma, corticosteroids are also used in the treatment of other inflammatory conditions such as eczema (as creams and ointments), rheumatoid arthritis (as injections) and in patients undergoing organ transplants. Usually found in a beige or brown inhaler, a number of different inhaled corticosteroids are now available for the control of asthma. These include beclometasone (Becotide®), budesonide (Pulmicort®), fluticasone (Flixotide®) and mometasone (Asmanex®).

Risks associated with corticosteroids

Corticosteroids are powerful drugs. In the past, the prolonged use of inhaled corticosteroids over periods of many years, has been linked to stunted linear (upwards) growth in children. Other side-effects that have been linked with the long-term use of high-dose corticosteroids include:

- fattened (or moon) face
- weight gain
- sudden mood swings
- easy bruising
- brittle bones (osteoporosis)
- cataracts in the eyes.

It is generally agreed that the risks associated with using corticosteroids are not as dangerous as living with asthma that is not properly controlled. The risk of experiencing any of these side-effects is very small, provided that corticosteroids are taken within the recommended guidelines.

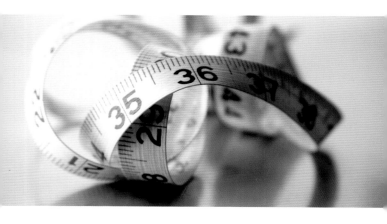

In the short-term, inhaled corticosteroids have also been associated with candidiasis of the mouth (a minor fungal infection). Using a spacer device, gargling with water or brushing your teeth after using corticosteroids can help to reduce the risk of infection.

If you have any concerns regarding the use of corticosteroids in children and teenagers, you should discuss them with your doctor.

Leukotriene receptor antagonists

A relatively recent addition to asthma therapy, the leukotriene receptor antagonist, montelukast (Singulair®), prevents inflammation of the airways by blocking the effects of leukotrienes. In contrast to other asthma treatments, montelukast is a chewable tablet, and in children, is available as granules (which can be taken directly or mixed with soft foods). Montelukast may be used in conjunction with inhaled corticosteroids to help prevent asthma attacks.

THE RELIEVERS

Relievers (also called bronchodilators) are drugs that quickly reverse the narrowing of the airways that occurs during an asthma attack.

A receptor is a structure inside or on the outside of a cell that binds to a specific substance and causes a specific biological effect.

Also known as bronchodilators, the relievers act by relaxing the muscle in the walls of the airways, which becomes tightened during an asthma attack. Relievers are also referred to as β_2-agonists (short for β_2-adrenoreceptor) in recognition of the drug receptor in the airways that they act on (see Simple Science).

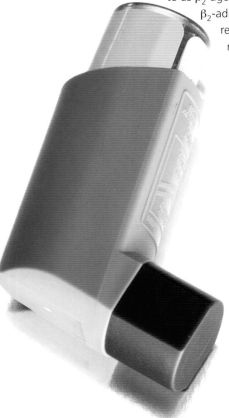

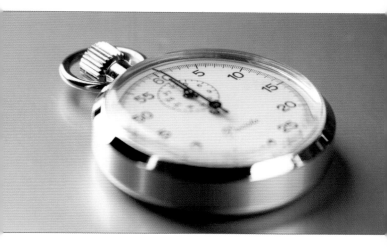

Short-acting β₂-agonists

Salbutamol (Ventolin®) and terbutaline (Bricanyl®) are short-acting β₂-agonists. Used on an 'as-needed' basis, these drugs get to work within minutes and quickly bring asthma symptoms under control. The beneficial effects of these drugs last for about 4 or 5 hours. They are usually found in a blue or grey inhaler. Everyone with asthma should have these inhalers available for occasional use. In cases of severe or life-threatening asthma, short-acting β₂-agonists can be rapidly administered via a nebuliser.

Long-acting β₂-agonists

Salmeterol (Serevent®) and formoterol (Foradil®, Oxis®) are long-acting β₂-agonists. These drugs act in much the same way as the short-acting β₂-agonists, except their effects last for up to 12 hours instead of 5. For this reason, long-acting β₂-agonists are particularly useful in the treatment of asthma symptoms that occur at night because they can control symptoms long enough for you to have a whole night of uninterrupted sleep. Long-acting β₂-agonists are used regularly, usually twice daily, in conjunction with inhaled corticosteroids (and can sometimes be administered in the same inhaler).

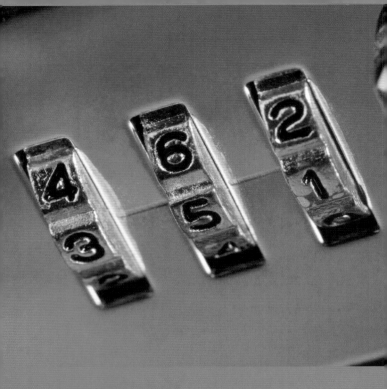

Preventer–reliever combinations

For many people with asthma, remembering to take their preventer medication on a regular basis can be difficult. The more inhalers there are to remember, the more confusing asthma medication can become, which can mean that you forget to take your inhaler and make yourself more likely to have an asthma attack. To solve this problem and improve convenience, some drug companies have produced combination inhalers which contain both a long-acting β_2-agonist and an inhaled corticosteroid. Seretide® (which contains salmeterol and fluticasone) and Symbicort® (which contains formoterol and budesonide) are examples of combination inhalers.

THE DIFFERENT TYPES OF ASTHMA MEDICATION

Generic name	Brand name	R/P?	Formulation
Beclometasone	Becotide®	P	Dry powder inhaler or aerosol
Budesonide	Pulmicort®	P	Dry powder inhaler or aerosol
Budesonide–Formoterol	Symbicort®	R/P	Dry powder inhaler or aerosol
Ciclesonide	Alvesco®	P	Aerosol inhaler
Fluticasone	Flixotide®	P	Dry powder inhaler or aerosol
Fluticasone–Salmeterol	Seretide®	R/P	Dry powder inhaler or aerosol
Formoterol	Foradil®, Oxis®	R	Dry powder inhaler
Mometasone	Asmanex®	P	Dry powder inhaler
Montelukast	Singulair®	P	Chewable tablets or granules
Salbutamol	Ventolin®	R	Dry powder inhaler or aerosol
Salmeterol	Serevent®	R	Dry powder inhaler or aerosol
Terbutaline	Bricanyl®	R	Dry powder inhaler or aerosol

P, preventer; R, reliever; R/P, dual mechanism of action.

Drugs often have more than one name. A generic name, which refers to its active ingredient, and a brand name, which is the trade name given to it by the pharmaceutical company. Salbutamol is a generic name and Ventolin® is a brand name.

SUMMARY OF THE MOST COMMONLY USED ASTHMA MEDICATIONS

Class	Drug (brand name)	How it works
Short-acting β_2-agonist	Salbutamol (Ventolin®) Terbutaline (Bricanyl®)	Bronchodilator (relaxes airway smooth muscle).
Long-acting β_2-agonist	Salmeterol (Serevent®) Formoterol (Foradil®, Oxis®)	Bronchodilator (relaxes airway smooth muscle).
Inhaled corticosteroids	Beclometasone (Becotide®) Budesonide (Pulmicort®) Fluticasone (Flixotide®) Mometasone (Asmanex®)	Prevents inflammation of the airways.
Leukotriene receptor antagonist	Montelukast (Singulair®)	Blocks the inflammatory effects of leukotrienes.
Methylxanthines	Theophylline (Nuelin SA®, Slo-Phyllin®, Uniphyllin Continus®)	Bronchodilator (relaxes airway smooth muscle).
Cromoglicates	Sodium cromoglicate (Intal®, Cromogen Easi-breathe®), nedocromil sodium (Tilade®)	Prevents asthma attacks.
Inhaled corticosteroid and β_2-agonist	Budesonide plus formoterol (Symbicort®), fluticasone plus salmeterol (Seretide®)	Prevents inflammation of the airways and helps to relax airway smooth muscle.

How quickly it works	Major side-effects
Rapidly (within 30 minutes). Lasts 4–6 hours.	Tremor, palpitations, rapid pulse, headache. May become less effective with continued use.
Rapidly. Lasts up to 12 hours.	Tremor, palpitations, rapid pulse, headache. May become less effective with continued use.
Maximum effects reached within days. Must be taken regularly for long-term control of asthma.	Short-term: oral fungal infection, sore throat. Long-term: bruising, osteoporosis, slowed growth rate.
Maximum effects reached within hours. Given as a tablet.	Headache, dry mouth, gastric upset, serious skin rash (rarely).
Usually reserved for the treatment of severe asthma. Given as a tablet.	Rapid pulse, palpitations, nausea, gastric upset.
Second choice preventer treatment after inhaled corticosteroids. Of questionable benefit.	Headache, nausea, vomiting, coughing, sore throat.
Both types of drug are contained in one handy inhaler.	The same as those for the individual constituent drugs.

YOUR INHALER

The majority of asthma medications are administered through inhalers. This method of delivery helps to ensure that drugs are deposited directly into the lungs so that they can start working as quickly as possible. Of course, there are a number of different types of inhaler available on the market, each with their own advantages and disadvantages. Some inhalers are unique to a particular type of drug. There are two main types of inhaler: **metered dose inhalers** (MDI) and **dry powder inhalers** (DPI).

It is very important that you learn how to use your inhaler properly. Your doctor or asthma nurse will be able to show you how and may check your technique from time to time.

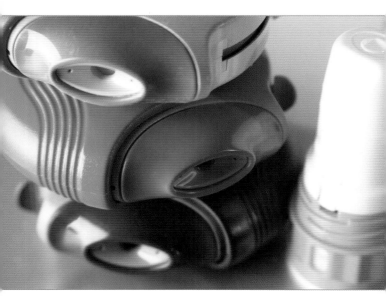

Metered dose inhalers

Metered dose inhalers use a propellant to 'fire' the drug into the lungs. In the past, the propellant was often a mixture of chlorofluorocarbon (CFC) gases but environmental concerns have prompted the introduction of non-CFC propellants. The guidance below sets out the best way for you to use your metered dose inhaler:

1 Shake the inhaler vigorously.

2 Remove the cap from the inhaler.

3 Check that the mouthpiece is clear of any dirt or foreign objects that you might otherwise inhale.

4 Stand up or sit up straight and breathe out.

5 Close your mouth around the end of the mouthpiece.

6 Breathe in slowly, and as you do so, push down on the top of the inhaler.

7 Continue to breathe in slowly for several seconds.

8 Hold your breath for as long as is comfortable, or up to 10 seconds.

9 Breathe out slowly.

10 Rinse your mouth with water or brush your teeth.

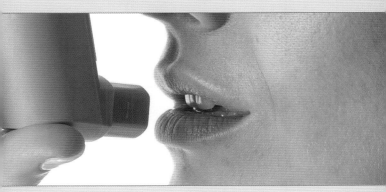

Dry powder inhalers

In dry powder inhalers, the drug is in powder, rather than aerosol, form. These devices require more effort to force the drug into the lungs, because there is no propellant to help you. For this reason, dry powder inhalers may also be called breath-actuated inhalers. Dry powder inhalers do not require the timing and co-ordination that are essential with metered dose inhalers. There are many types of dry powder inhaler. Some have to be loaded each time they are used, whilst others are preloaded with a fixed number of doses. Directions for use vary between inhalers, so it is important you ask your doctor or pharmacist about brand-specific instructions before using your inhaler. The following guidelines may help.

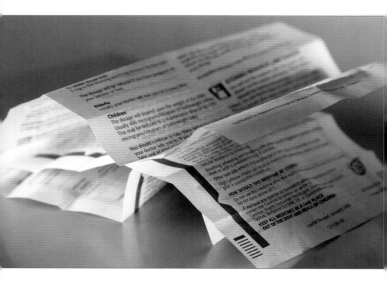

1 Do not shake the inhaler. Remove the cap and hold the inhaler upright.

2 Check that the mouthpiece is clear of any dirt or foreign objects that you might otherwise inhale.

3 Load a dose into the inhaler according to its accompanying instructions.

4 Tilt your head back slightly, and breathe out slowly. Take care not to breathe into the inhaler because the moisture in your breath may clog the mechanism.

5 Close your mouth around the end of the mouthpiece.

6 Breathe in quickly and deeply.

7 Remove the inhaler from your mouth.

8 Hold your breath for as long as is comfortable, or up to 10 seconds.

9 Breathe out slowly.

10 If you need to take a second inhalation, it is important that you wait for 30 seconds before doing so.

11 Rinse your mouth with water or brush your teeth.

Spacer devices

Spacers are used with metered dose inhalers to help direct the asthma medication into the lungs, and thereby prevent it from depositing in your mouth. As mentioned previously, inhaling corticosteroids on a regular basis can lead to candidiasis, a fungal infection of the mouth. Although this is not by any means life-threatening, it is not particularly pleasant. Spacers can be detachable plastic tubes (obtained without prescription from your pharmacy) or are sometimes built into the inhaler. Depending on the device, the following guidance may be useful.

1 Fit the inhaler to the inhaler hole in the spacer device.

2 Put the mouthpiece of the spacer in your mouth or put the mask over your nose and mouth.

3 Spray the asthma medicine into the spacer once.

4 Take a deep breath and hold it for 10 seconds.

5 Breathe out into the spacer.

6 Repeat two or three times with the mouthpiece still in your mouth.

7 Never spray the two puffs into the spacer together as it is not nearly as effective as doing them separately.

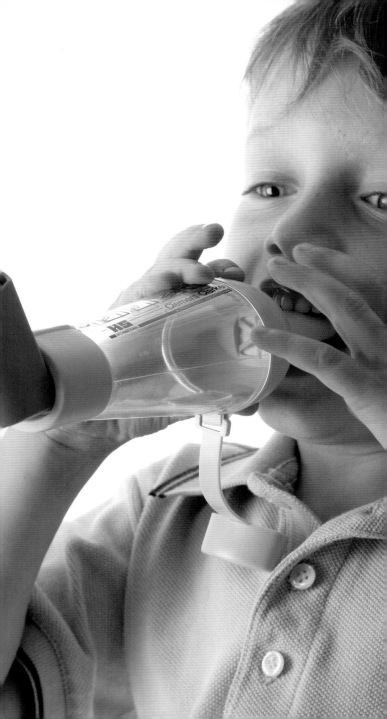

Inhalers and children

The British Thoracic Society (BTS) has recommended that children under the age of 5 use a metered dose inhaler with a spacer attachment (and a face mask if necessary). If this is ineffective, a nebuliser may be used. Younger children may find it easier to use a dry powder inhaler.

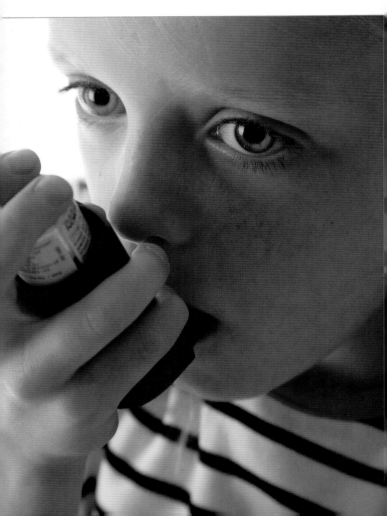

NEBULISERS

Nebulisers are devices that pump air or oxygen through a liquid medicine to turn it into a vapour, which is then inhaled by the patient.

Nebulisers provide quick relief of asthma symptoms and are most commonly used to treat severe attacks of asthma at a doctor's surgery or in an A & E department in the case of an emergency.

Usually, the nebuliser will be a small plastic container that is filled with a solution of drug. A compressor (usually electric) is used to bubble air or oxygen through this solution to make a fine mist of medicine. This mist is breathed into the lungs through a mouthpiece or face mask.

A person with asthma will not usually have their own nebuliser. They are expensive, often bulky and are difficult to keep clean. For the majority of people, an inhaler is the most practical drug delivery device.

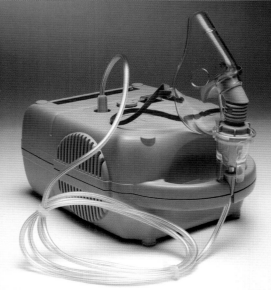

89

SOURCE: CLEMENT CLARKE INTERNATIONAL LIMITED.

A 'STEPWISE' TREATMENT APPROACH

After consulting with you, your asthma management team will design an asthma management programme that fits in with your specific needs. To help them, specific guidelines have been issued by the British Thoracic Society (BTS) and the National Institute for Clinical Excellence (NICE), and these strongly recommend a 'stepwise' approach to treatment. This means that asthma treatment is initiated at the lowest stage that is necessary to control your asthma adequately. If the treatment at one stage is not working, your doctor may recommend moving you up to the next step. Conversely, if your asthma is well controlled, your doctor may recommend moving your treatment down a step.

Stepping down is when a patient moves from more intensive to less intensive drug treatment.

You should ask your doctor if you are concerned about any aspect of your asthma treatment. Patients may respond in slightly different ways to the same medicine. If you experience symptoms which you think may be due to the medication you are taking, you should talk to your doctor, pharmacist or nurse. If the side-effect is unusual or severe, your GP may decide to report it to the Medicines and Healthcare Products Regulatory Agency (MHRA). The MHRA operates a 'Yellow Card Scheme' which is designed to flag up potentially dangerous drug effects and thereby protect patient safety. The procedure has changed recently to allow patients to report adverse drug reactions themselves. Visit *www.yellowcard.gov.uk* for more information.

Consider the various steps of drug treatment like the rungs of a ladder. Following diagnosis, you will be started on the lowest rung of the ladder, only progressing to the next rung up (and the next strength of medication) if your asthma is not controlled sufficiently. As you work your way up the ladder, the side-effects associated with drug treatment become more severe, so it is important to stay on the lowest rung that controls your asthma. When you reach a rung at which your asthma is controlled, over time, your GP may decide to 'step down' your medications, so that you remain on the lowest possible dose of drug.

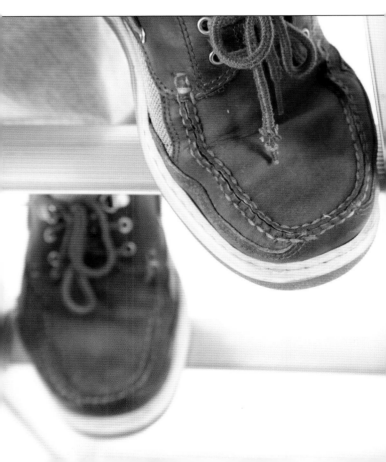

Rung 1

You occasionally use a reliever. If you are regularly using it more than once a day or once at night your treatment should move up to the next rung.

Rung 2

In addition to your reliever, you may now need to take regular preventer treatment to reduce the inflammation in your airways. At this stage, this will usually be a low-dose corticosteroid inhaler.

Rung 3

If your asthma is not fully controlled, your doctor will offer you an 'add-on therapy'. The first add-on therapy to be tried is usually a long-acting reliever, taken in addition to your corticosteroid preventer. Your symptoms will then be reassessed to see if there has been an improvement. At this stage, it may also be necessary to increase your dose of inhaled steroid, with the agreement of your GP. There are other add-on treatments available (e.g. montelukast) and if the long-acting reliever medicine has no effect, your doctor should stop this treatment before introducing other types of medication.

Rung 4

In addition to your long-acting reliever medicine (if it is helping to reduce your symptoms),the dose of your steroid inhaler medicine may be increased further. Other add-on therapies may be introduced if your symptoms are difficult to control.

Rung 5

If your symptoms are still not under control, even on maximum amounts of medication, you may be referred to a respiratory specialist. You may be started on a course of steroid tablets.

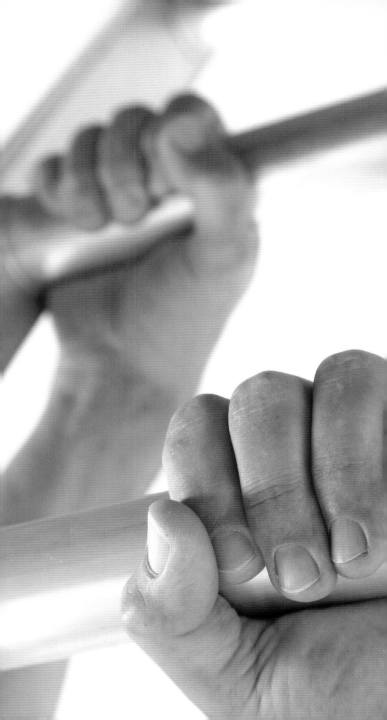

ASTHMA IN CHILDREN

Treating asthma in children involves a slightly different approach to that taken in adults. Although the overall 'ladder' of control follows the same general pattern, the doses of drugs used to treat children will be significantly lower than those used to treat adults. As a parent, you may be concerned about side-effects related to certain asthma treatments, but be assured that your GP will try to use the lowest dose of drug possible to control your child's symptoms. The lower the dose, the less likely your child is to get side-effects. Ask your doctor if you are concerned about any aspect of your child's treatment.

Another important difference between adults and children is exactly who assumes the responsibility for asthma control. Since, generally speaking, children are less capable of taking control of their asthma, this usually falls to the parent or caregiver. You should make sure that your child carries their inhalers with them at all times, and try to keep track of any changes in their symptoms.

ASTHMA AT SCHOOL

It is important that you ensure your child's teachers are aware that they have asthma. Many schools will have asthma management policies in place to make sure children with asthma receive the care and attention they need.

■ Make sure the school knows that your child has asthma.

■ Clearly explain which medications your child is on and when they must be taken.

■ Make sure your child has free access to their reliever medication.

■ Ensure that teachers are aware of your child's personal asthma triggers.

■ Ensure that the teachers know how to deal with an asthma attack.

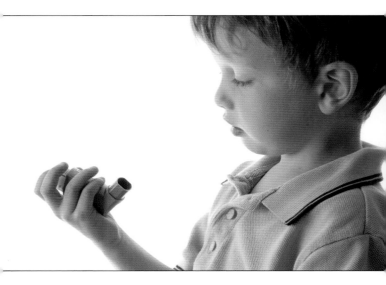

MANAGING ASTHMA DURING PREGNANCY

Usually, you will not need to change your asthma medication whilst you are pregnant.

Being pregnant can affect the severity of your asthma. Some women may find that their asthma gets worse, whilst others may notice no difference in their symptoms at all. It is also extremely important that you inform your obstetrician that you have asthma. If you have concerns about asthma and pregnancy, you may wish to ask the following questions.

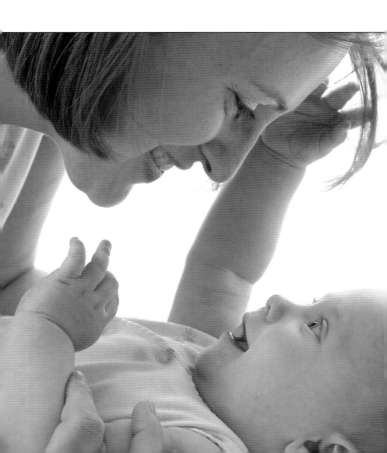

- What complications may occur if I don't take my medication?
- What complications may occur if I do take my medication?
- Will my baby get enough oxygen if I am short of breath?
- What kind of labour should I plan to have?
- Should I have an epidural?
- Will my medication affect my baby if I choose to breast feed?
- Is it likely that my baby will have asthma too?

It is particularly important that you do not smoke whilst you are pregnant, because this may have repercussions for your unborn child.

It is important that women with asthma who are pregnant, or who are intending to become pregnant, seek medical advice from their GP or a member of their asthma management team. They will recommend that your asthma is monitored regularly over the course of your pregnancy.

ALTERNATIVE TREATMENTS FOR ASTHMA

Complementary, or alternative, treatment can play an important role in the long-term management of asthma. However, it should never replace the conventional asthma medication prescribed for you by your doctor. You should always keep your asthma management team informed of any alternative medication or techniques you are using to control your asthma, in case these interfere with the programme of care he/she is recommending.

Complementary medicine is often belief-based rather than evidence-based.

Although alternative therapies can be very effective, and many people swear by them, the main reason that they are not recommended as 'stand-alone' methods of controlling asthma is that the clinical evidence to back them up is often lacking. Claims regarding their effectiveness and safety are generally not reinforced by well-designed clinical trials performed with lots of people. This is in stark contrast to asthma drugs, which have to go through strict testing procedures before they can be widely used in patients.

Some of the most popular alternative means of controlling asthma are described below. These include homeopathy, acupuncture and yoga. There are a number of complementary medicine organisations nationally (see Simple Extras) and your GP may even be able to put you in touch with some of these.

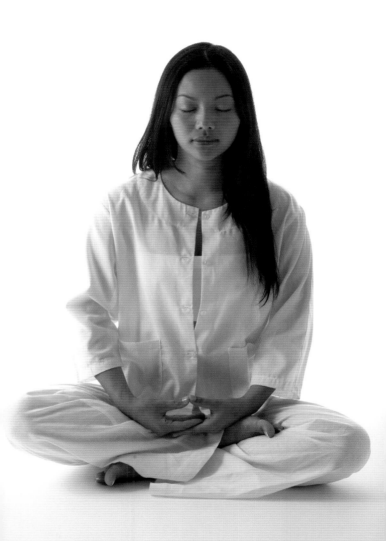

COMPLEMENTARY THERAPY FOR ASTHMA

The Buteyko technique

A system of breathing exercises and behavioural changes intended to improve health by altering the balance of oxygen and carbon dioxide in the air you breathe out. Very little information has been published in medical journals about the effectiveness of the Buteyko technique.

Yoga

Pranayama yoga, a variety of postures and breathing techniques to help to increase fitness and aid relaxation, has been studied with regard to asthma. Some exercises were found to be beneficial, with patients showing fewer asthma attacks and a higher tolerance to certain triggers.

Hypnosis

May be beneficial in some people with asthma, but not everybody is susceptible to hypnosis.

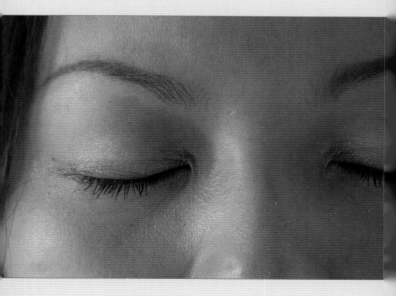

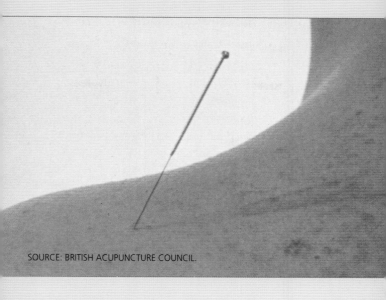

SOURCE: BRITISH ACUPUNCTURE COUNCIL.

Acupuncture

Involves the insertion of needles at specific points on the body, and is based on Chinese theories of balancing the body's natural energies. Some studies have shown that acupuncture can be helpful for people with asthma in the short term. However, no long-term benefits have yet been shown and more research is needed before it can be universally recommended.

Homeopathy

Homeopathy may be helpful in asthma if the allergic trigger can be identified, but this is not always easy as most people have more than one trigger. Although some research has shown homeopathy to be helpful in asthma, more research is needed in larger groups of people.

THE LONG AND THE SHORT OF IT

Is asthma life-threatening?

Fewer people die from asthma than used to be the case. Compared with years gone by, the number of asthma-related deaths has decreased dramatically, and this is probably as a result of better treatments and management approaches. Although more than 1,400 people still die from asthma in the UK each year, it has been estimated that up to 90% of these deaths are preventable, given proper treatment and management.

Will it go away on its own?

Generally speaking, if you develop asthma as an adult it will probably remain with you for the rest of your life. Some children will grow out of their asthma, whilst others won't. At the moment, there is no way of telling who will and who won't.

The most important thing is not to ignore the symptoms of asthma. By doing so you are placing yourself at unnecessary risk.

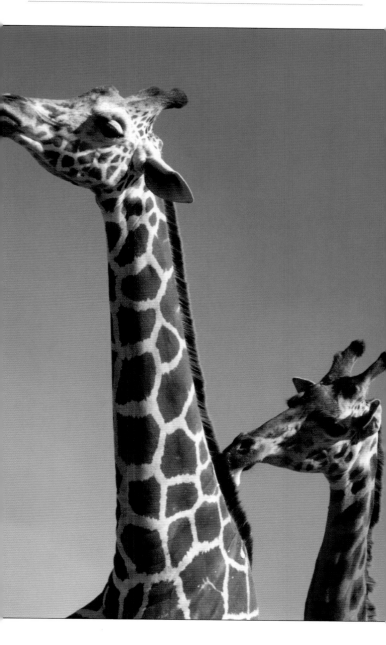

BECOMING AN EXPERT PATIENT

Asthma is a long-term disease that usually affects you for the rest of your life. People with asthma may benefit from joining the Expert Patient Programme, run by the NHS. The scheme is aimed at encouraging people with long-term health conditions to take more control over their health by understanding and managing their conditions. By enrolling on the Expert Patient Programme you will ultimately be able to use your skills and knowledge to lead a fuller life. Courses take 6 weeks to complete and are run throughout the country. Visit *www.expertpatients.nhs.uk* for more information.

You may find the 6-Point Asthma Patient Self-Assessment Checklist a useful means of measuring how well your asthma (or allergic rhinitis) is controlled. Find it at www.allergyuk.org

GETTING THE MOST OUT OF YOUR HEALTH SERVICE

Asthma is a long-term condition that needs to be treated on a case-by-case basis. Maintaining a good relationship with your GP, or any other member of your asthma management team, is fundamental to managing your asthma effectively. This involves effort from both sides. You should keep them informed of your symptoms on a regular basis and conversely, they should dedicate sufficient time and effort to managing your asthma.

It is important to have regular review appointments with a member of your asthma management team to monitor both your asthma symptoms and the treatment you are taking. Most surgeries now provide dedicated 'asthma clinics', where a full asthma assessment is made by a trained asthma nurse or GP. You should visit your surgery every 6 months, or more regularly if you have just been diagnosed with asthma.

There is good evidence that people who have regular checks have fewer asthma attacks, less time off work and enjoy a better health-related quality of life. For people who are unable to get to the surgery for check-ups, telephone asthma checks may be useful and many surgeries now provide this facility. Most importantly, if you have any questions, surrounding any aspect of your asthma, don't be afraid to ask.

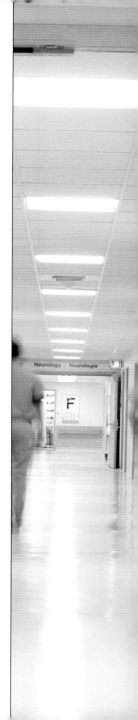

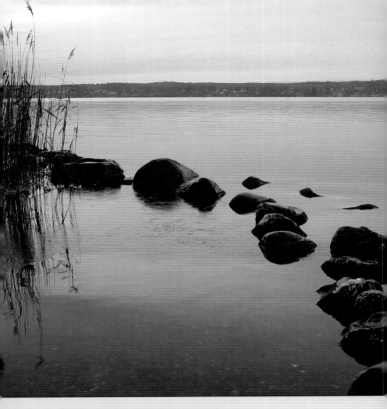

QUESTIONS TO ASK YOUR DOCTOR

- How do you know for certain that I have asthma?
- Why do I have asthma?
- How severe is my asthma?
- Will my asthma get worse?
- How often should I come in for check-ups?
- What type of treatment suits me best?
- When should I use my reliever and when should I use my preventer?
- What will happen if I do take my medication?
- What will happen if I don't take my medication?
- What is the correct way to use an inhaler?
- Should I be using a spacer with my metered dose inhaler?
- What should I do if my asthma gets worse suddenly?
- How can I learn more about my asthma?

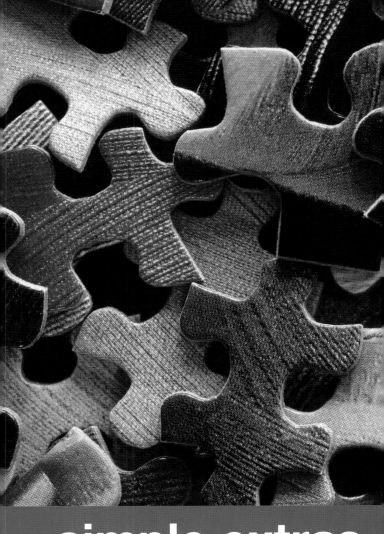

simple extras

FURTHER READING

■ *BESTMEDICINE Asthma* (2005)
CSF Medical Communications Ltd, Oxford
320 pp, ISBN: 1-905064-94-2, £13.95
Website: *www.bestmedicine.com*

■ **British Guideline on the Management of Asthma (2003)**
British Thoracic Society and Scottish Intercollegiate Guidelines
Network (SIGN)
Websites: *www.brit-thoracic.org.uk*
www.sign.ac.uk

USEFUL CONTACTS

■ **Action on Smoking and Health (ASH)**
102 Clifton Street
London
EC2A 4HW
Email: *enquiries@ash.org.uk*
Tel: 020 7739 5902
Website: *www.ash.org.uk*

■ **Allergy UK**
3 White Oak Square
London Road
Swanley
Kent
BR8 7AG
Allergy Helpline: 01322 619898
Tel: 020 8303 8525
Website: *www.allergyuk.org*
Email: *info@allergyuk.org*

■ **Asthma UK**
Summit House
70 Wilson Street
London
EC2A 2DB
Email: *info@asthma.org.uk*
Tel: 020 7786 4900
Asthma UK Adviceline: 08457 010203
Website: *www.asthma.org.uk*
Formerly called the National Asthma Campaign

■ **Asthma UK Scotland**
4 Queen Street
Edinburgh
EH2 IJE
Tel: 0131 226 2544
Email: *enquiries@asthma.org.uk*
Website: *www.asthma.org.uk*

■ **British Acupuncture Council**
63 Jeddo Road
London
W12 9HQ
Email: *info@acupuncture.org.uk*
Tel: 020 8735 0400
Website: *www.acupuncture.org.uk*

■ **British Lung Foundation**
73–75 Goswell Road
London
EC1V 7ER
Email: *enquiries@blf-uk.org*
Tel: 020 7688 5555
Helpline: 08458 50 50 20
Website: *www.lunguk.org*

British Thoracic Society
17 Doughty Street
London
WC1N 2PL
Email: *bts@brit-thoracic.org.uk*
Tel: 020 7831 8778
Website: *www.brit-thoracic.org.uk*

■ **General Practice Airways Group**
Smithy House
Waterbeck
Lockerbie
DG11 3EY
Email: *info@gpiag.org*
Tel: 01461 600639
Website: *www.gpiag.org*

■ **Global Initiative for Asthma (GINA)**
Website: *www.ginasthma.com*

■ **NHS Direct**
Website: *www.nhsdirect.nhs.uk*

■ **NHS Smoking Adviceline**: 0800 1690169

■ **Occupational Asthma**
Health and Safety Executive
Tel: 08701 545500
Website: *www.hse.gov.uk/asthma*

■ **The Patients Association**
PO Box 935
Harrow
Middlesex
HA1 3XJ
Helpline: 0845 608 4455
Tel: 020 8423 9111
Website: *www.patients-association.com*

YOUR RIGHTS

As a patient, you have a number of important rights. These include the right to the best possible standard of care, the right to information, the right to dignity and respect, the right to confidentiality and underpinning all of these, the right to good health.

Occasionally, you may feel as though your rights have been compromised, or you may be unsure of where you stand when it comes to qualifying for certain treatments or services. In these instances, there are a number of organisations you can turn to for help and advice. Remember that lodging a complaint against your health service should not compromise the quality of care you receive, either now or in the future.

- **Patients Association**
  The Patients Association (*www.patients-association.com*) is a UK charity which represents patient rights, influences health policy and campaigns for better patient care.
  Contact details:
  PO Box 935
  Harrow
  Middlesex
  HA1 3YJ
  Helpline: 08456 084455
  Email: *mailbox@patients-association.com*

- **Citizens Advice Bureau**
  The Citizens Advice Bureau (*www.nacab.org.uk*) provides free, independent and confidential advice to NHS patients at a number of outreach centres located throughout the country (*www.adviceguide.org.uk*).
  Contact details:
  Find your local Citizens Advice Bureau using the search tool at *www.citizensadvice.org.uk*

- **Patient Advice and Liaison Services (PALS)**
  Set up by the Department of Health (*www.dh.gov.uk*), PALS
  provide information, support and confidential advice to patients,
  families and their carers.
  Contact details:
  Phoning your local hospital, clinic, GP surgery or health centre
  and ask for details of the PALS, or call NHS Direct on 0845 46 47.

- **The Independent Complaints Advocacy Service (ICAS)**
  ICAS is an independent service that can help you bring about
  formal complaints against your NHS practitioner. ICAS provides
  support, help, advice and advocacy from experienced advisors
  and caseworkers.
  Contact details:
  ICAS Central Team
  Myddelton House
  115–123 Pentonville Road
  London N1 9LZ
  Email: *icascentralteam@citizensadvice.org.uk*
  Or contact your local ICAS office direct.

Accessing your medical records

You have a legal right to see all your health records under the Data
Protection Act of 1998. You can usually make an informal request to
your doctor and you should be given access within 40 days. Note
that you may have to pay a small fee for the privilege.

You can be denied access to your records if your doctor believes
that the information contained within them could cause serious
harm to you or another person. If you are applying for access on
behalf of someone else, then you will not be granted access to
information which the patient gave to his or her doctor on the
understanding that it would remain confidential.

PERSONAL RECORD:

My Simple Guide

This Simple Guide to Asthma belongs to:

Name:

Address:

Tel No:

Email:

In case of emergency please contact:

Name:

Address:

Tel No:

Email:

My Healthcare Team

GP surgery address and telephone number

Name: _____

Address: _____

_____

_____

Tel No: _____

I am registered with Dr _____

_____

My specialist asthma nurse _____

My respiratory specialist _____

My pharmacist _____

Other members of my healthcare team _____

_____

_____

_____

QUESTIONS

_____

_____

_____

_____

_____

_____

_____

_____

_____

_____

_____

_____

_____

_____

_____

ANSWERS

_____

_____

_____

_____

_____

_____

_____

_____

_____

_____

_____

_____

_____

_____

_____

_____

NOTES